Muscular Injuries in the Posterior Leg

J. Bryan Dixon
Editor

Muscular Injuries in the Posterior Leg

Assessment and Treatment

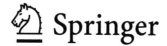

Springer

Editor
J. Bryan Dixon, MD
Sports Medicine
Advanced Center for Orthopedics
Marquette, MI, USA

ISBN 978-1-4939-7941-7   ISBN 978-1-4899-7651-2   (eBook)
DOI 10.1007/978-1-4899-7651-2

Springer Boston Heidelberg New York Dordrecht London
© Springer Science+Business Media New York 2016
Softcover reprint of the hardcover 1st edition 2016

Printed on acid-free paper

Springer US is part of Springer Science+Business Media (www.springer.com)

In memory of Dr. Bo Michael Rowan.

Preface

Recorded sports medicine dates to the advent of the Olympic Games. Scholars have suggested that Hippocrates himself learned his orthopedics from treating athletes. Sports injuries are unmistakable in the chiseled sculptures of ancient athletes—centuries of weathered wear still reveal the corpulent auricular hematoma of the grappler and saddle nose deformity of the pugilist. The notable absence of muscle injuries enshrined in marble reflects the devastating effect of muscle injuries on performance. The victor and veteran may be marred by their craft, but they must be fit to function in order to compete.

Like ancient Greece, we are seeing a modern resurgence of physical culture and a renewed appreciation for the intertwined nature of exercise and health. If exercise is medicine, then sports medicine is medicine sine qua non. As muscle is the engine of movement and movement is the basis for sport and health, then a detailed knowledge of muscle should be foundational to sports medicine. As sports medicine professionals, we must consider that muscle injuries are arguably the most important injuries for our patients' health and performance.

Muscles make up almost half of our bodies; it is the stratum of sport, a remarkable engine for our ingenuity. With muscles, we do, we move and react, we rally and retreat. In professional sport, we see the headlines reporting the sprinter laid low or pitcher lost from the lineup due to muscle injuries. But the greatest burden of muscle injuries is not found on the sports pages, rather it is the countless recreational athletes unable to run, cycle, and play basketball or soccer. This book is dedicated to the colossal toll muscle injuries have on physical activity and to the hobbled masses yearning to run free. Through a dedicated and detailed examination of muscle injuries of the posterior leg, I hope this book also provides a robust foundation to understand muscle injuries more generally.

Muscular injuries of the posterior leg have a rich history. Originally, it was termed "tennis leg," a reference to the lawn tennis of the 1800s, not the Wimbledon of the Williams sisters. Tennis leg is emblematic of modern sports injuries and perhaps the first sport-specific injury described in the medical literature. At one time, tennis leg prompted spirited investigation and professional debate, but the focus on muscular injuries has slowly faded, replaced by more glamorous injuries that are amenable to heroic treatments. Today, beyond the brief refrain of rest, ice, compression, and elevation (RICE) and rehab, little is found in medical texts about tennis leg or other muscle injuries.

Yet, muscle injuries continue to be a source of significant morbidity for our patients. Message boards and blogs abound with stories of patients suffering from the lasting effects of muscle injures and requests for help.

This book aims to put the focus back on muscle injuries, to restore the primacy and place of these widespread maladies, long displaced by the pathology popularized by our peers and in the press. Anterior cruciate ligament (ACL) tears and Tommy John's repairs represent the modern paradigm of sports medicine, and their treatment brings professional prestige and public notoriety, as evermore heroic treatments are performed by physicians utilizing novel procedures backed by remarkable technological innovation.

I think you will find that the optimal evaluation and treatment of muscle injuries has all the subtlety and gratification of the more heroically treated injuries that currently dominate sports medicine. Skeletal muscle is the paradigm for the biological structure–function relationship. At any scale, skeletal muscle intricately links structure and function. Appreciating this link between structure and function forms the basis for diagnosis, treatment, and prevention of muscle injuries. With increased knowledge of the basic science of muscle and muscular injuries, we are entering a new era of understanding and innovative treatment options.

It is time to revisit our roots to acknowledge and appreciate the tremendous consequence muscle injuries have on athletes and active people, to take back professional pride in the thoughtful treatment of muscular malfunction, and to collaborate and not delegate the care of this important class of injuries. Your interest in this book shows you care about muscle injuries and I commend your commitment to learning more about these failures of the flesh. I know from experience that your commitment will be rewarded by thankful patients and excited collaborators in treatment of these injuries. I welcome your feedback on this book or specific questions on the optimal care of your patients. I look forward to joining you in future discussion and investigations on the assessment, treatment, and prevention of muscular injuries.

Marquette, MI   J. Bryan Dixon, MD

Contents

Contributors

Morhaf Al Achkar, MD Clinical Family Medicine, Indiana University—Methodist Hospital, Indianapolis, IN, USA

John Baldea, MD Clinical Family Medicine, Indiana University School of Medicine, Family Medicine IU Health, Indianapolis, IN, USA

Julia C. Bisschops, MD, MSc Sports Medicine Institute, Family Medicine Department, Memorial Hospital, South Bend, IN, USA

Jeffrey S. Brault, DO Department of Physical Medicine and Rehabilitation, Mayo Clinic, Rochester, MN, USA

Conan Von Chittick, MD Family Medicine/Sports Medicine, IU Health Methodist Hospital, Indianapolis, IN, USA

Casey Chrzastowski, DPT Outpatient Orthopedics, Rehabilitation Services, IU Health West, Avon, IN, USA

Manoj K. Dhariwal, MD Millennium Physician Group, Port Charlotte, FL, USA

J. Bryan Dixon, MD Sports Medicine, Advanced Center for Orthopedics, Marquette, MI, USA

Scott N. Drum, PhD ACSM-CES, CSCS, FACSM School of Health and Human Performance, Northern Michigan University, Marquette, MI, USA

Christopher Robert Faber, MD Emergency Department, Baraga County Memorial Hospital, L'Anse, MI, USA

Stacey M. Hall, PT, MS Physical Therapy, Indiana University Health, Indianapolis, IN, USA

Premod John, MD Department of Family Medicine, IU Methodist Hospital, Indianapolis, IN, USA

Christopher C. Jordan, MD AT Sports Medicine, Saint Joseph Regional Medical Center, Mishawaka, IN, USA

Mark E. Lavallee, MD, CSCS, FACSM Sports Medicine Institute, Family Medicine Department, Memorial Hospital, South Bend, IN, USA

Zachary C. Leonard, MD Orthopedic Surgery, Advanced Center for Orthopedics, Marquette, MI, USA

Brock McMillen, MD Clinical Medicine, Family Medicine, Indiana University School of Medicine—IU Methodist Hospital, Indianapolis, IN, USA

Erich N. Ottem, PhD Department of Biology, Northern Michigan University, Marquette, MI, USA

Jeremy L. Riehm, DO Medical Education, Saint Joseph Regional Medical Center, Mishawaka, IN, USA

Bo M. Rowan, DO Marquette Family Medicine Residency Program, DLP Marquette, Marquette, MI, USA

Stephen M. Simons, MD, FACSM Sports Medicine, Saint Joseph Regional Medical Center, Mishawaka, IN, USA

Eric P. Sturos, MD Department of Physical Medicine and Rehabilitation, Vanderbilt University School of Medicine, Nashville, TN, USA

Andrew Swentik, MD Orthopedic Surgery, University of South Carolina, Columbia, SC, USA

Ryan Weatherwax, MS Department of Recreation and Exercise and Sport Science, Western State Colorado University, Gunnison, CO, USA

Jordana Weber, MD Family Medicine, Methodist Hospital, Indianapolis, IN, USA

Ryan R. Woods, MD Department of Physical Medicine and Rehabilitation, Mayo Clinic, Rochester, MN, USA

Part I

Underlying Principles in the Assessment and Treatment of Muscular Injuries of the Posterior Leg

Anatomy of the Leg

1

Julia C. Bisschops and Mark E. Lavallee

The Skeletal Structures of the Leg

The leg is part of the lower extremity and specifically the region of the body between the knee and ankle. Often the lower extremity is inaccurately called the leg, but the leg is only one of the six major regions of the lower extremity, including the gluteal region (hip and buttocks), thigh, knee, leg, ankle, and foot. The leg consists of two bones: the tibia and the fibula. As limb bones, they are part of the appendicular skeleton and are classified as long bones. They are covered in a sleeve of periosteum that provides neurovascular support to the bone and deposition of new bone after trauma or chronic stress. The periosteum also serves a critical role in linking soft tissue elements to bone.

The tibia is the main weight-bearing support structure. It transfers weight and force from the knee to the ankle and determines the shape of the leg. The fibula, found lateral and posterior to the tibia, does not articulate with the femur and is largely non-weight bearing [1]. The tibia and fibula are firmly connected by the interosseous membrane, which at the terminal ends is also called the syndesmotic ligament. The fibers of the interosseous membrane run distal and

lateral from the tibia to the fibula connecting at the lateral crest of the tibia to the anteromedial border of the fibula [2]. This thick strong membrane keeps the two bones held together tightly, aiding in stabilization of the ankle and providing additional stability for attachment of the muscles of the leg. In addition to the interosseous membrane, the tibia and fibula are connected by joints both superiorly and inferiorly.

The tibia itself consists of a metaphyseal region, an epiphyseal region, and an articular surface that is made of hyaline cartilage. Its most proximal end forms the inferior surface of the knee joint and is called the tibial plateau; more specifically, the proximal tibia is divided into three parts: medial and lateral plateaus and tibial eminence. The tibial eminence consists of two parts: medial and lateral tibial spines (they are also called lateral and medial intercondylar tubercles) as seen in Fig. 1.1 [3]. Specifically, this area consists of an anterior intercondylar area and a posterior intercondylar area. This structure is of importance because it is where the anterior cruciate ligament (ACL), posterior cruciate ligament (PCL), and medial and lateral menisci attach [2]. Just distal to the articular surface of the tibial plateau and located near the lateral condyle of the tibia is a fibular facet that articulates with the proximal fibula to form the superior joint connecting the two bones. On its anterior surface, the tibia has a tuberosity, which marks the end of the epiphyseal line and is distal to the attachment of the patella tendon. The attachment for the iliotibial band is located on the proximal part of the

J. C. Bisschops (✉) · M. E. Lavallee
Sports Medicine Institute, Family Medicine Department,
Memorial Hospital, South Bend, IN, USA
e-mail: JBisschops@beaconhealthsystem.org

M. E. Lavallee
e-mail: mlavallee@wellspan.org

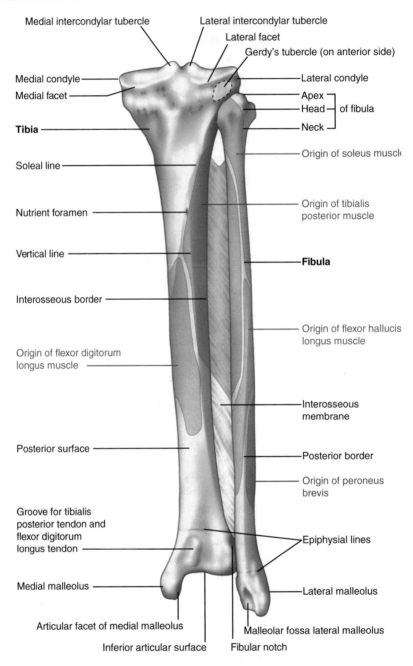

Fig. 1.1 This drawing shows the two major bones of the lower extremity: the *tibia* and the *fibula*. It gives an overview of all the different structures located on these two bones, mostly focused on the *posterior surface*. In addition, origins of muscles are labeled to illustrate where the major muscles of the posterior lower leg originate

anterolateral tibia and is called Gerdy's tubercle [2]. It was named after the French surgeon and anatomist Pierre Nicolas Gerdy, whose name has also been associated with a number of other anatomical structures [4].

The shaft of the tibia consists of a medial, a lateral, and a posterior surface. The anteromedial surface of the tibia or "shin" is subcutaneous and easily palpated in most people. Whereas the anteromedial part of the tibia has virtually no attachments, the posterior part has a significant number of attachments: semimembranous, popliteus, soleus, tibialis posterior, and flexor digitorum longus (the vertical line separates the two latter muscles). The posterior surface of the tibia includes muscular attachments relevant to muscular injuries of the posterior leg. In general, the flexor muscles are attached to the posterior part of the tibial shaft [2]. The posterior surface is bound by the interosseous and medial borders of the tibia. Both the soleal line and the vertical line are located on the posterior surface. The distal end of the tibia articulates with the fibula and talus to form the ankle joint. The distal tibia consists of a number of different surfaces: anterior, medial, posterior, lateral, and distal. The most distal aspect of the tibia is the medial malleolus, just lateral to this is the groove for the tibialis posterior tendon.

Running posterolateral to the tibia, the fibula is the thinner and weaker of the two leg bones. The fibula does not articulate with the femur and has a limited role in weight bearing. It is the site of the distal muscular attachment of the biceps femoris and muscular origin of several muscles of the leg. It begins proximally at the fibular head, an easily palpated structure found just posterolateral to the lateral tibial plateau. The fibula head is an important landmark because this is the location to which a number of clinically significant structures attach: extensor digitorum longus and peroneus longus and soleus, as well as the fibular collateral ligament, or lateral collateral ligament (LCL), connected to the biceps femoris. Below the head, the fibula consists of a shaft and the lateral malleolus, also known as the distal end of the fibula. The shaft has three surfaces and borders: anterior, posterior, and interosseous. The posterior surface is the largest of these and includes muscular attachments for the tibialis posterior, soleus, flexor hallucis longus, peroneus longus, and peroneus brevis, while the anterior surface includes attachments for the extensor digitorum longus and extensor hallucis longus [3]. Please see Fig. 1.1 for illustration of the mentioned bony structures and attachments.

Soft Tissue Structures of the Leg

In the leg, as throughout the limbs, functionally related groups of muscles are contained in fascial compartments. These compartments are bound by a thick canvas-like covering of deep fascia and share a neurovascular supply. The soft tissues of the leg are divided into four of these compartments: the anterior, the lateral, the superficial posterior, and the deep posterior. These four compartments are divided by crural (leg) fascia, also called fascia cruris, which is the deep fascia of the lower leg; more posterior, it is known as the popliteal fascia.

Although the main focus of this book is on the muscles of the superficial and the deep posterior compartments, the proximity of the lateral and posterior compartments as well as their functional overlap necessitates careful delineation of lateral and posterior compartments clinically. The lateral compartment houses several clinically important structures, including the common peroneal nerve, the peroneus longus, and the peroneus brevis. The peroneus longus is the more superficial of the two muscles; it everts and plantarflexes the foot (Fig. 1.2) [3].

The most distal part of this peroneus longus consists of a very long tendon. The peroneus brevis is located just anterior to the peroneus longus. The common peroneal nerve moves from its proximal posterior location behind the fibular head to an anterior lateral position as it transverses between the fibular head and shaft. Both muscles are supplied by the superficial peroneal nerve, which also provides sensory innervation to the dorsum of the foot.

The superficial posterior compartment consists of the gastrocnemius, soleus, plantaris, and tendo calcaneus (Achilles tendon) . As a functional unit, the superficial posterior compartment is critical in maintaining functions of standing posture and gait. As a group, they primarily assist in flexing the knee and plantarflexing the foot.

The gastrocnemius is the largest and most superficial muscle of the superficial posterior compartment. Its heart-shaped landmarks are easily visible through the skin in well-trained athletes. The more proximal part of the gastrocnemius (its

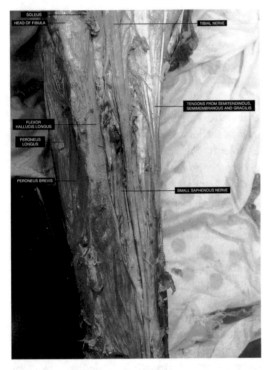

Fig. 1.2 This picture, taken in the anatomy laboratory, illustrates the location of the *peroneus longus* and the *peroneus brevis* muscles and their location in relation to the fibula and some of the other structures of the posterior leg such as the *soleus* and the *tibial nerve*

"belly") originates from two heads, which are connected to the femoral condyles by tendons. More specifically, there is a medial and a lateral head. The medial head tends to be the larger of the two. On its distal end, the muscle becomes narrower and blends to form a union with the Achilles tendon. Starting above the knee and extending beyond the ankle to the calcaneus, the gastrocnemius crosses two joints. This biarthodial architecture conveys a unique functional continuity with the hamstrings in initiating knee flexion and limiting knee extension. Rarely, individuals may not have a lateral head of the gastrocnemius, or a third head may be present [5]. The tibial nerve provides the innervation of the gastrocnemius.

The soleus, located just deep or anterior to the gastrocnemius, is a broad and flat muscle. The soleus has a central tendon and pennate structure. Unlike the gastrocnemius, which spans two joints (the knee and the ankle), the soleus originates

on the posterior tibia and crosses only the ankle joint. It is attached proximally to the posterior border of the tibia and fibula by an arch-like aponeurosis with a tendinous gap centrally. The posterior tibial artery and tibial nerve pass through this gap to enter the deep posterior compartment. The more distal end of the muscle connects to the gastrocnemius, which then, as noted above, forms the Achilles tendon. As a result, there is a strong synergistic relationship between the gastrocnemius, the soleus, and the Achilles tendon, which is important in regard to the injuries discussed in the following chapters. Please see Figs. 1.3 and 1.4 for illustration of the mentioned muscles.

The soleus has a high percentage of fatigue-resistant muscle fibers and plays a critical role in maintaining standing posture and walking gait. The soleus muscle is supplied by two branches of the tibial nerve. Accessory soleus muscles are well-known but uncommon congenital anomaly [6]. An accessory soleus can be a source of exertional pain due to an inadequate blood supply from the posterior tibial artery.

The plantaris is a rather small muscle and actually has been found absent in a number of individuals. It originates from the lateral supracondylar line deep to the lateral head of the gastrocnemius. From this lateral attachment on the femur, it moves medial as it extends distal. The muscle ends shortly after crossing the knee joint, where at approximately the origin of the soleus, it transitions in a long, thin tendon that traverses between the medial head of the gastrocnemius and the soleus before inserting on the medial calcaneus either independently or by means of the Achilles tendon. In the setting of an Achilles tendon rupture and a preserved independent attachment of the plantaris tendon to the calcaneus, the ability to plantarflex the ankle can remain potentially confounding for the clinical diagnosis. The plantaris is supplied by the tibial nerve. It is referred to by some as the gastrocnemius's "little helper," as it acts in conjunction with the gastrocnemius in an accessory fashion. Like the gastrocnemius, it crosses both the knee and ankle but due to its small size and absence in some individuals, the functional role of the plantaris is tradition-

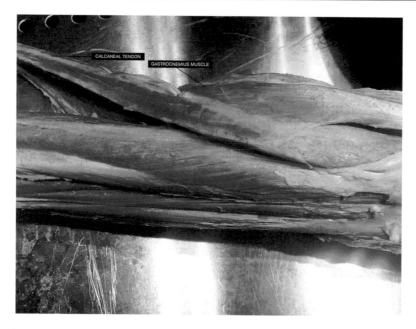

Fig. 1.3 Another picture taken in the anatomy laboratory illustrating the strong relationship between the *gastrocnemius muscle* and the *calcaneal tendon*

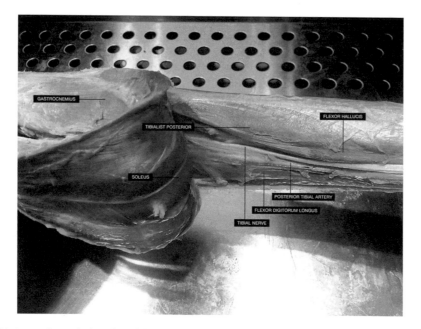

Fig. 1.4 This image shows the location of the *soleus,* a broad and flat muscle, found deep to the *gastrocnemius*. In addition, the *tibial nerve* is labeled, innervating both the *gastrocnemius* and the *soleus*

ally thought to be relatively insignificant and it is considered by many to be a vestigial muscle. Indeed, the plantaris tendon is harvested for autograph tendon repair for this very reason [7].

However, the pattern of a small muscle running in parallel with a larger prime mover has been termed parallel muscle combination, and in these combinations the small muscle has been found

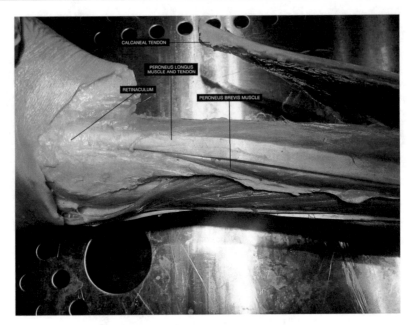

Fig. 1.5 This picture, again taken in the anatomy laboratory, shows the lateral side of the right leg. It shows the *peroneus longus muscle* and the *peroneus brevis muscle* and the largest human tendon, the *calcaneal tendon*, which has been cut. The *retinaculum* is a structure that wraps around a number of vessels, nerves, and muscles of the lower leg as they enter the foot. It will be mentioned again later in this chapter

to have a high density of muscle spindles. Some authors have proposed these muscles may serve an important proprioceptive function, providing neurologic feedback to regulate movement [8]. It should be noted that discussion regarding the function of the plantaris can be influenced by larger arguments regarding the implications of vestigial muscle as evidence for evolution [9].

The tendo calcaneus or calcaneal tendon or, more commonly, Achilles tendon, another member of the posterior superficial compartment, is the shared tendon insertion of the gastrocnemius, soleus, and plantaris. It is the largest human tendon and its thickness makes it the strongest tendon in the body, a feature critical to its importance during running gait where it must handle loads up to ten times the body weight. It begins as a wide, flat apponerous formed from the myotendinous junction of the gastrocnemius, soleus, and plantaris. As it descends, it narrows and thickens, its fibers spiraling downwards like a tree root, conferring additional mechanical advantage and improved storage of energy in eccentric loading,

to attach securely along the periosteum of the heel and directly into the calcaneus. These structural features of the Achilles tendon are critical in function of the human gait (Fig. 1.5).

The vascular supply to the Achilles tendon is fed both proximally and distally by the posterior tibial artery, leaving the midsubstance of the tendon in a watershed area of relative hypovascularity supplied by the peroneal artery [10–12]. The midsubstance of the Achilles tendon is the most common location for degenerative tendinopathy and Achilles tendon ruptures. Innervation of the Achilles tendon comes from both the sural and tibial nerves [13].

The superficial and the deep compartments are separated by deep transverse fascia, located between the medial tibial and the posterior fibular borders. The deep posterior compartment, often also called the deep crural group, consists of deep transverse fascia, popliteus, flexor hallucis longus, flexor digitorum longus, and tibialis posterior. The popliteus is a flat, triangular muscle, found deep and at the most distal part of the popliteal fossa. Its innervation is supplied by the tibial nerve. The popliteus helps rotate the tibia medially, or rotate the femur laterally if the tibia is fixed or in a "closed-chain" position. Due to its connections, it is believed to aid the PCL to prevent forward motion of the femur. The flexor hallucis longus is supplied by the tibial nerve (please see earlier images). Flexor digitorum longus, found medial to the flexor hallucis longus, is also innervated by the tibial nerve. Both of these flexors act on the distal phalanges. The tibialis posterior is found between the flexor hallucis longus and the flexor digitorum longus and is partially covered by both of these muscles [3]. At the distal end it passes deep to the flexor retinaculum (as visible in the previous image). The tibialis posterior is also innervated by the tibial nerve. It is responsible for inverting the foot and aids in plantar flexion. It is also known to aid in balancing and controlling pronation.

The tendons of many of the muscles mentioned eventually cross the talocrural (ankle) joint. They are covered by a number of retinacula: superior extensor, inferior extensor, flexor, peroneal, and a number of synovial sheaths (part of these may be visualized in the mentioned images). Theoretically, these structures are part of the foot, but part of the leg structures pass through them, so they are mentioned for understanding and completion. Most notable is the flexor retinaculum because it is directly connected to the medial calcaneal process and plantar aponeurosis. The posterior vessels and nerve enter here, as well as the tibialis posterior, flexor digitorum longus, and flexor hallucis longus, all previously mentioned [3].

The Vascular Supply of the Leg

The main vascular structure feeding the lower extremity is the popliteal artery. This artery divides into three branches, more specifically, the anterior tibial artery, the posterior tibial artery, and the peroneal artery. We will focus on the posterior tibial artery and the peroneal artery. The peroneal artery is also called the fibular artery and can be a branch of the posterior tibial artery.

The posterior tibial artery starts at the most distal border of the popliteus. This artery can be found between the tibia and the fibula. Distally, it divides into the medial and lateral plantar arteries. It is palpable medial to the medial malleolus. On its way, it gives off the following branches: circumflex fibular (may also arise from the anterior tibial artery), peroneal, nutrient, and the medial and lateral plantar arteries (already mentioned) [3]. The circumflex fibular artery wraps around the fibulas neck, as its name suggests. Its vulnerable locations make it more prone to trauma. The peroneal artery, also called the fibula artery, originates distally to the popliteus muscle. It runs more laterally compared to the posterior tibial artery. Generally, it runs between the tibialis posterior and the flexor hallucis longus. As it is about to reach the calcaneus, it divides into the calcaneal branches. A number of anatomical variations have been found. Some of these variations can give rise to popliteal artery entrapment syndromes resulting in exertional lower leg pain. More specifically, the peroneal artery, at times, may originate more distally from the posterior tibial artery. The following arteries are branches from the peroneal artery: small muscular branches that help supply some of the posterior-compartment muscles, a nutrient artery to the fibula, a perforating branch serving the interosseous membrane, either one or two communicating branches between the posterior tibial artery and the peroneal artery, and the already-mentioned calcaneal branches [3]. Please see Fig. 1.6 for an overview of some of these structures.

The above description mentions two nutrient arteries, one that supplies the tibia and one that helps supply the fibula. It is worth mentioning that most of the human tibia is supplied by this single nutrient artery as it enters through a nutrient foramen, usually in the more proximal part of the tibia. The external surface of the tibia is only covered by a periosteum, again supplied by the nutrient artery. This anatomical fact explains why injury and trauma around the tibial area are quite difficult to heal [2].

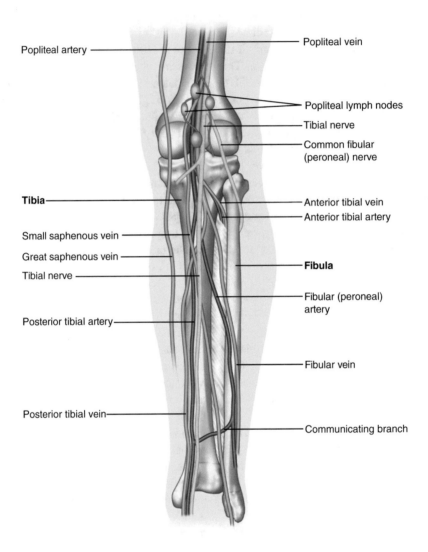

Fig. 1.6 This drawing shows the posterior right leg. It gives an overview of the arteries, veins, and nerves of the lower extremity. Also, the location of the *popliteal lymph nodes,* as mentioned in the text, is visualized here

Venous System of the Posterior Leg

In general, two sets of veins drain the lower extremities: the superficial veins and the deep veins. The deep veins often accompany arteries. Both sets of veins have valves that limit backflow. The venous valves, deep fascia, and contraction of the muscle within the leg compartments work in concert to return blood to the heart, a process termed the musculovenous pump.

The superficial veins consist of the great/long saphenous vein and the small/short saphenous vein. Both have numerous smaller branches, many of them unnamed. The great saphenous vein is the longest vein in our body, ending into the femoral vein. Along its journey, it has a number of accompanying nerves, such as the saphenous nerve, meeting the nerve around the tibiomalleolus area. The small saphenous vein runs more laterally as it passes between the heads of the gastrocnemius and eventually empties into

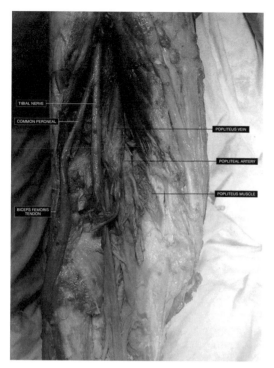

Fig. 1.7 This picture illustrates part of the popliteal fossa. It shows the previously mentioned *popliteus muscle* and the *popliteal vein* and *artery*. The *biceps femoris tendon* originates in the upper leg but attaches here as illustrated

the popliteal vein. Numerous connections exist between smaller branches and the great saphenous and small saphenous veins [3].

The deep veins of the leg mainly comprise the posterior tibial vein, the anterior tibial vein, the popliteal vein, the femoral vein, and, for completion purposes, the vena profunda femoris. The posterior tibial vein accompanies the posterior tibial artery. The anterior tibial vein forms the popliteal vein. More distally, it runs between the tibia and the fibula. The popliteal vein runs medially to the popliteal artery. The femoral vein runs together with its artery [3]. Please see Fig. 1.7 for an illustration of some of these deep structures.

Lymphatic Drainage

Superficial and deep are the recurrent themes of lower extremity anatomy, and this also holds true for the lymphatic drainage of the leg. More specifically, lymph nodes are found at the follow-

ing locations in the lower extremity: superficial inguinal nodes, deep inguinal nodes, and popliteal lymph nodes. Focus will be on the popliteal lymph nodes, since they are located in the posterior leg. Around six lymph nodes are found in the popliteal area. They ascend either into the deep inguinal nodes or, occasionally, into the superficial inguinal nodes. Injuries and infections in lower extremity areas such as the heel would lead to swelling of the popliteal nodes. Medial and lateral lymphatic vessels drain superficial tissues, while the deep lymphatic vessels drain the deep tissues to the popliteal nodes as mentioned earlier (see Fig. 1.6) [3].

Nerves of the Leg

The two main nerves in the leg are the tibial nerve and the common peroneal nerve, also called fibular nerve, as illustrated in Fig. 1.8.

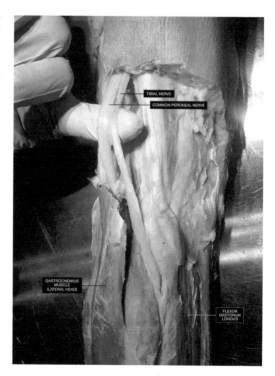

Fig. 1.8 This photograph points out the size and location of the main nerves of the leg: *tibial* and *common peroneal* (fibular nerve). In addition, the *lateral head* of the gastrocnemius may be visualized

Both nerves originate from the sciatic nerve, which originates from the sacral plexus. The tibial nerve is usually the bigger of the two. It is located deep in its proximal location, but quite superficial as it passes through the flexor retinaculum (see Fig. 1.5). More specifically, it runs with the posterior tibial vessels, first medial to them and then lateral. It has a number of branches: articular, muscular, sural, medial calcaneal, and medial/lateral plantar [3]. The lateral plantar nerve has one specific branch that is of importance, due to frequent involvement in entrapment leading to discomfort and injury in athletes—the Baxter's nerve. It is usually the first branch of the lateral plantar nerve and runs through the porta pedis, where if entrapped, causes discomfort.

The common peroneal nerve, also called fibular nerve or lateral popliteal nerve, is much smaller than the tibial nerve. It runs on the lateral side of the popliteal fossa. When it wraps around the head of the fibula, it becomes palpable. This is the location where it is most prone to injury, and injury to this nerve often results in foot drop. It innervates the peroneus longus and brevis muscles. The common peroneal nerve can be further divided into auricular and cutaneous branches. Its auricular branch accompanies the superior and inferior lateral genicular arteries; the third auricular branch is the recurrent articular nerve, which accompanies the anterior recurrent tibial artery. The cutaneous branches are called the lateral sural nerve, also known as the lateral cutaneous nerve of the calf, and the sural communicating nerve. The common peroneal nerve may further be divided into the deep peroneal nerve, also called anterior tibial nerve, and the superficial peroneal nerve, also called musculocutaneous nerve. The deep peroneal nerve descends with the anterior tibial artery to the ankle. The superficial peroneal nerve supplies the peroneus longus, brevis, and skin of the lower leg. Both of the mentioned nerves may be subdivided even further. The deep peroneal nerve divides into a muscular branch, a lateral terminal branch, a medial terminal branch, an articular branch to the ankle joint, and an interosseous branch. The superficial peroneal nerve communicates with a number of nerves and has a smaller lateral and medial branch [3]. The sural,

saphenous, common peroneal, superficial peroneal, and deep peroneal nerves can all develop clinically relevant entrapment syndromes.

The posterior lower limb can roughly be divided into four cutaneous (dermatome) nerve distributions: superficial to the popliteal fossa: posterior cutaneous of thigh S1,2,3; just lateral to popliteal fossa: medial cutaneous of thigh L2,3; superficial to medial gastrocnemius: saphenous L3,4; and lateral gastrocnemius: lateral cutaneous of calf of leg L4,5,S1.

Acknowledgments The authors acknowledge the contribution of IU/Notre Dame Anatomy Laboratory.

References

1. Marx JA. Marx: Rosen's emergency medicine. 7th ed. Philadelphia: Mosby Elsevier; 2010.
2. Browner BD. Browner: skeletal trauma. 4th ed. Philadelphia: Saunders Elsevier; 2009.
3. Williams PL, Warwick R. Gray's anatomy. 37th ed. London: Churchill Livingstone; 1989.
4. Beals TC. So who was Gerdy … and how did he get his own tubercle? Am J Orthop. 1996;25(11):750–2.
5. Yildirim FB, et al. The co-existence of the gastrocnemius tertius and accessory soleus muscles. J Korean Med Sci. 2011;26:1376–81.
6. Brodie JT, Dormans JP, Gregg JR, Davidson RS. Accessory soleus muscle. A report of 4 cases and review of the literature. Clin Orthop Relat Res. 1997;337:180–6.
7. Daseler EH, Anson BJ. The plantaris muscle: an anatomical study of 750 specimens. J Bone Jt Surg. 1943;25:822–7.
8. Peck D, Buxton DF, Nitz A. A comparison of spindle concentrations in large and small muscles acting in parallel combinations. J Morphol. 1984;180(3):243–52.
9. Menton D. The plantaris and the question of vestigial muscles in man. J Creation. 2000;14(2):50–3.
10. Chen TM, Rozen WM, Pan WR, Ashton MW, Richardson MD, Taylor GI. The arterial anatomy of the Achilles tendon: anatomical study and clinical implications. Clin Anat. 2009;22(3):377–85.
11. Matusz P. About the arterial anatomy of the Achilles tendon (tendo calcaneus). Clin Anat. 2010;23(2):243–4. (Author reply 245).
12. Theobald P, Benjamin M, Nokes L, Pugh N. Review of the vascularisation of the human Achilles tendon. Injury. 2005;36(11):1267–72. (Epub 2005 Apr 19).
13. Doral MN, Alam M, Bozkurt M, Turhan E, Atay OA, Dönmez G, Maffulli N. Functional anatomy of the Achilles tendon. Knee Surg Sports Traumatol Arthrosc. 2010;18(5):638–43. (Epub 2010 Feb 25).

Physiology of Skeletal Muscle

Scott N. Drum, Ryan Weatherwax and J. Bryan Dixon

Introduction

Skeletal muscle is necessary for every movement of the human body. The physiology of skeletal muscle is the foundation for understanding human movement and muscle injuries. Skeletal muscle has one primary task; namely, to transform chemical energy into mechanical energy. Simply stated, muscle converts the chemical energy of our diet into fuel for muscle action and then, when stimulated by the nervous system, skeletal muscle uses this fuel to produce mechanical energy in the form of muscle action.

In this chapter, we review each of these components of skeletal muscle physiology and how they relate to practical applications in nutrition, rehabilitation, and sport. We begin with metabolism and the process of skeletal muscle energetics. The details of the skeletal muscle machinery and control of muscular action are the focus of the remaining sections of this chapter.

S. N. Drum (✉)
School of Health and Human Performance, Northern Michigan University, Marquette, MI, USA
e-mail: sdrum@nmu.edu

R. Weatherwax
Department of Recreation and Exercise and Sport Science, Western State Colorado University, Gunnison, CO, USA

J. B. Dixon
Sports Medicine, Advanced Center for Orthopedics, Marquette, MI, USA
e-mail: jbryandixon@hotmail.com

Metabolism

Macronutrient Use, ATP Production, and Energy Pathways

In order to fully appreciate the physiology of skeletal muscle, you must know how muscle transforms the food we eat into the muscular action that produces force and motion. This flow of energy is called skeletal muscle energetics and it focuses on the creation and use of adenosine triphosphate (ATP). ATP is the energy currency of the body. In skeletal muscle, ATP is responsible for contraction and relaxation of skeletal muscle.

Skeletal muscle energetics begins with macronutrient consumption. When ingesting macronutrients, we start to convert food into energy—a process called metabolism. Macronutrients, such as a combination of carbohydrate, fat, and protein, are reduced to their basic form primarily of glucose, fatty acids, and amino acids, respectively, when used in metabolic processes to produce ATP, the energy currency of the body. Importantly, glucose and fatty acids are used more commonly than protein for sustained muscular action. This preserves protein and its constituent amino acids as the building blocks of skeletal muscle. Because protein serves in a lesser capacity as energy precursor, the focus of skeletal muscle energetics is on carbohydrate and fats.

To more clearly understand how macronutrients promote the production of ATP and subsequent performance in various activities, such as endurance exercise, let us consider a classic study [1]. In this experiment, participants were fed a high-fat diet (5% or less carbohydrate intake), normal diet (met the recommended daily allowance of carbohydrate, lipid, and protein), and a high-carbohydrate diet (82% of calories from carbohydrates). When tested in a repeated-measures design, all subjects underwent all feeding conditions for 3 days with recovery days in between conditions and bouts on a cycle ergometer to exhaustion. Not only did the high-carbohydrate diet produce the best glycogen storage (i.e., stored glucose in skeletal muscle that was six times greater than the high-fat diet), but time to exhaustion when cycling was also three times longer than the high-fat diet. The normal diet fell in between. Therefore, when thinking about optimizing endurance performance, carbohydrate stored in skeletal muscle and even in the liver is paramount to sustaining high-intensity muscular actions, especially when exercising or competing longer than 1 h. Other studies have since supported this [2, 3].

On the other hand, high-fat *meals* may help boost endurance exercise as well, but only as long as an adequate carbohydrate *diet* is followed. For instance, ingesting a high-fat *meal* (1007 ± 21 kcal/meal in total calories; 30% carbohydrates, 55% fat, and 15% protein) 4 h before an exercise bout after 3 days of a high-carbohydrate *diet* (2562 ± 19 kcal/day in total calories: 71% carbohydrates, 19% fat, and 10% protein) and with tapered training, demonstrated the greatest time until exhaustion versus ingesting a high-carbohydrate *meal* (1007 ± 21 kcal, 71% CHO, 20% F and 9% P) after the 3 days of high-carbohydrate intake [4]. Interestingly, just prior to exercise, in the high-fat meal group, participants ingested a maltodextrin jelly or placebo. In the high-carbohydrate meal condition, participants ingested only a placebo. From a practical viewpoint, the above study underscored the need for sufficient carbohydrate intake prior to exhaustive exercise to maintain strong skeletal muscle action with the addition of a high-fat meal showing some benefit. Thus, skeletal muscle macronutrient needs during sustained muscular action are nicely supported by both carbohydrate and fat, with a preference for carbohydrate as the exercise intensity increases. This is excellent information to remember in view of optimizing skeletal muscle physiological properties. Note that because high-intensity, short-duration exercise is usually much less than 1 h, a reliance on carbohydrate is the norm with almost no risk of glycogen depletion.

The production of ATP from various macronutrients follows three primary energy pathways that use various substrates (e.g., carbohydrate, fat, phosphocreatine (PCr), among others) to produce ATP. These energy pathways, from fastest to slowest rate of ATP production, are: (1) ATP-PCr or phosphagen, (2) glycolytic or lactic acid, and (3) aerobic processes [5]. Said another way, these three energy-producing pathways are preferentially favored during differing durations of intense exercise of approximately 0–15 s, 16–90 s, and >90 s, respectively. Keeping these pathways and associated timeframes in mind during the following discussion about skeletal muscle physiology, helps maintain a helpful perspective on human performance.

On elaborating individual energy pathways, we find that, in short, the ATP-PCr pathway, or "fast" ATP-producing process, utilizes a coupled reaction in the cytoplasm whereby the breakdown of PCr by creatine kinase to creatine (C) + inorganic phosphate (P_i) yields energy used to synthesize ATP from the recombination of adenosine diphosphate (ADP) + P_i. The glycolytic system, also housed in the cytoplasm and a "fast" ATP-producing process that may be described as anaerobic or aerobic, relies mostly on glucose degradation from blood or stored skeletal muscle glycogen with the end products of lactic acid (which spontaneously becomes lactate + H^+ if anaerobic ATP production is favored) and/or pyruvic acid (which spontaneously becomes pyruvate if aerobic ATP production is feasible). To summarize, if exercise is "slow" or low intensity in nature, then pyruvate production is favored whereas, the buildup of lactate + H^+ in tissue and blood occurs when exercise is "fast" or high intensity. Not surprisingly, various glycolytic enzymes, some rate limiting, control the glycolytic process and are namely: hexokinase

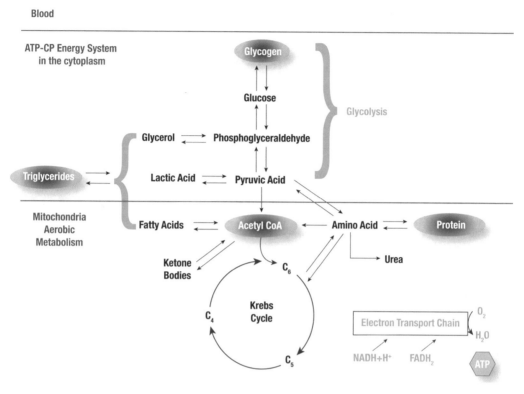

Fig. 2.1 The interaction of carbohydrates, triglycerides, and proteins, termed macronutrients, in the metabolic pathway. Note that all macronutrients have the capability to become Acetyl CoA, the common entryway to the oxidative energy cycle. Likewise, each macronutrient has the potential to become a different substrate in the metabolic process. Thus, metabolic precursors are highly interrelated. (Courtesy of Elizabeth A. Drum)

(HK), phosphofructokinase (PFK), and lactate dehydrogenase (LDH).

The aerobic energy system takes place in the mitochondrion of a skeletal muscle cell and begins when pyruvate (from aerobic glycolysis) is converted to Acetyl CoA and combines with oxaloacetate (OOA) within the organelle as part of the Krebs or citric acid cycle [5]. Both carbohydrate and fat (with negligible input from protein sources) are utilized at rest and during exercise, depending on intensity (i.e., low to moderate), to "run" aerobic processes. ATP creation, also known as oxidative phosphorylation, occurs in the electron transport chain (ETC) via H$^+$s shuttled from the Krebs cycle to the ETC via electron shuttles (i.e., nicotinamide adenine dinucleotide, NAD$^+$; and flavin adenine dinucleotide, FAD). Therefore, ATP is synthesized by transferring electrons from NADH and FADH$_2$ to oxygen in the ETC [5]. Keep in mind that as a person

exercises on a regular basis, more mitochondria, denser muscle mass, improved blood flow, and greater aerobic (and anaerobic) enzymes are upregulated. With cessation of exercise these changes reverse. Figure 2.1, below, depicts the interaction of the aforementioned energy pathways and the use of carbohydrates, fats, and proteins in the metabolic synthesis of ATP.

Muscle Fiber Types

Having reviewed macronutrient utilization in skeletal muscle cells in accordance with energy pathways to produce ATP for sustained muscular action, we now transition to a discussion of muscle fiber types. Skeletal musculature is composed of slow- and fast-twitch (ST and FT, respectively) fibers or cells. ST are also known as type I or slow-oxidative (SO) cells and rely

Table 2.1 Skeletal muscle/fiber classification

System 1	Type I	Type II	Type IIx
System 2	Slow twitch (ST)	Fast twitch a (FTa)	Fast twitch x (FTx)
System 3	Slow oxidative (SO)	Fast oxidative/glycolytic (FOG)	Fast glycolytic (FG)
General attributes of fiber types			
Oxidative ability	Excellent	Good	Poor
Glycolytic ability	Poor	Excellent	Excellent
Contractile speed	Slow	Fast	Fast
Fatigue resistant	Excellent	Good	Poor
Unit strength	Poor	Excellent	Excellent

primarily on the aerobic energy system to produce ATP for muscle action. FT fibers, also known as type II fibers, are further categorized as FTa and FTx or type IIa and type IIx, respectively. FT fibers rely more on the ATP-PCr and anaerobic glycolytic energy pathways to sustain high intense action with a high rate of ATP production.

In general, type II muscle fibers are larger, transmit action potentials faster, have greater activity of the ATP splitting enzyme myosin ATPase, release and uptake calcium ions (Ca^{2+}) more rapidly, and exhibit a high-rate crossbridge turnover (between actin and myosin or skeletal muscle myofibrils) than type I fibers, which exhibit all the aforementioned characteristics albeit at a protracted rate. Additionally, type II fibers tend to store more carbohydrate and are favored during high-intensity and/or power-strength exercises. Type I fibers, on the other hand, favor aerobic or low- to moderate-intensity exercise and rely on both carbohydrate and fat as fuel (note, both of these macronutrients are stored in type I fibers). Additionally, type I fibers have a greater concentration of mitochondria and capillaries versus type II fibers [5]. See Table 2.1 for a side by side comparison of the various fiber types.

Skeletal Muscle Force Production

We have seen that skeletal muscle physiology creates the opportunity for a plethora of muscle actions based on the combination of fiber types and energy pathways available. With the varied pathways to manufacture ATP, there is balance between low-energy requirements (e.g., rest or low-moderate-intensity exercise) and high-energy needs (e.g., high-intensity exercise). Notably, skeletal muscle can be selectively recruited to the muscular action needed based on fiber type and/or size of the fibers. Generally, as alluded above, type I fibers are smaller and therefore innervated by smaller alpha motor neurons, the primary neurons responsible for initiating muscular action. The size principle implies that during force development of progressively increasing magnitude, type I fibers are recruited first, followed by type IIa, and finally type IIx, the most powerful fiber set [6].

Therefore, the discussion about force production begins with acknowledging that the process of developing force in muscle is efficiently regulated, especially by increasing motor unit recruitment and increasing the frequency of motor unit discharge [5]. Recognize that a motor unit is, by definition, a single motor neuron and all the fibers it innervates—from a few to thousands [5]. The following section introduces the properties of skeletal muscle that allow it to exert force, namely the sliding filament theory (SFT). Underlying the mechanics of force production are the omnipresent metabolic processes that maintain the ATP supply for sustainable muscle action and, therefore, force output. Said another way, you get work (W) output, which equals force (F) times distance (D) or $W = F \times D$. This is a useful equation to remember when discussing muscular force production in that internal muscular force normally equals an external result, such as the movement of a weight stack or self-propulsion during walking or running.

A Few Muscle Action Definitions

A muscle fiber contraction or shortening of the muscle belly is a complex process that involves cellular and chemical interactions. The result is movement within the myofibrils in which thin (actin) and thick (myosin) filaments slide past and over one another. A muscular action may cause a shortening of a sarcomere, the smallest contractile unit of a muscle fiber, under tension (and ultimately a shortening of the muscle or contraction). This is termed as concentric muscle action. When the filaments slide in a direction causing a lengthening of the sarcomere under tension, an eccentric muscle action is created. When concentric and eccentric muscle actions are performed continuously, one after the other, such as during a full range of motion movement during a bench press exercise using free weights, this is termed isotonic exercise. Isometric muscle action, another relatable term, is created when thick and thin filaments attempt to slide in either direction, but a fixed or static length is held for a period of time. In other words, there is no lengthening or shortening of the sarcomere in a static action, even though energy is continuously being utilized to fuel the isometric event; maintaining your posture while sitting is a good example of static torso action. Another pertinent muscle movement to mention is isokinetic action in which muscle fibers exert a near constant, maximal force throughout a preset constant speed as seen in the use of an isokinetic Cybex machine in the rehabilitation setting.

Collectively, all the muscular actions mentioned above provide a brief overview of how specificity in resistance training methods can be incorporated with the principle of overload to create a thoughtful training or rehabilitation plan. Taken together, overload is the progressive increase in resistance on a particular muscle group over time in a systematic and specific fashion to elicit muscular force application and adaptation changes. Discussion of the role of resistance training in rehabilitation and performance training plans is covered in the later chapters of this book.

Sliding Filament Theory (SFT)

Working independently in 1954, H. E. Huxley [7] and A. F. Huxley [8] were involved in establishing the SFT. The theory explains how fixed-length thick (myosin) and thin (actin) filaments move in relation to each other, resulting in a change in muscle length and subsequently force production. In 1957, A. F. Huxley [9] further elaborated this model with a theory of crossbridge behavior which offered insights into how muscular force application is accomplished via internal, microscopic force application mechanisms. We have already established that metabolically force cannot be produced and sustained without macronutrient- or substrate-derived ATP. This primary energy structure is what interacts with muscle fiber myofilaments, actin and myosin, to allow the sliding filament model to "run" and crossbridge formation to unfold. Force happens when muscular action occurs (either concentric or eccentric). However, neurological input, discussed later in this chapter, is necessary to the initiation of muscle action via Ca^{2+} release into the sarcoplasm via specific structures. With that in mind, we turn to a few more characteristics of muscular force generation before returning to a more detailed discussion of the SFT.

Types of Muscular Action Relationships

Having introduced the SFT, where microscopic force application occurs, let us discuss a bit more about types of muscular interactions. Keep in mind that the term contraction can be misleading when discussing muscle properties and force-generating capabilities. Contraction of skeletal muscle seems to denote primarily a shortening of the fibers. However, in this chapter, we want to underscore that it indicates a shortening, lengthening, retention of the same length, or a combination of these depending on external loads and the desired activity. Therefore, a muscular *contraction* more accurately reflects a muscular action, than a contraction per se. Following are a few muscle fiber relationships that will help round out a review of muscular force production or the lack thereof.

Length–Tension Relationship

The length of a muscle fiber relative to its optimal length is critical in determining the amount of force or tension that can be developed. The optimal length can be defined as the length of the sarcomere, the smallest contractile unit of a fiber, that provides ideal overlap of thick and thin filaments [10]. Therefore, when optimal length is obtained in a sarcomere, normally around 90° in a joint, the greatest amount of force production is possible because of optimal actin–myosin interaction. Hence, when a muscle is shorter or longer than *optimal* length, there is impairment in maximal or optimal force production. For additional information concerning this type of relationship, especially in active muscle, the reader is directed to review Rassier et al.'s paper [11] titled *Length dependence of active force production in skeletal muscle*. Figure 2.2, below, illustrates various knee angles and the angular position that elicit the greatest muscular tension or strength.

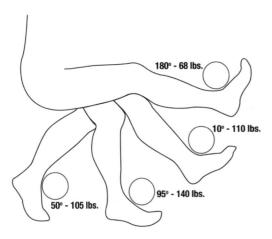

Fig. 2.2 Length–tension relationship of various joint angles, such as the knee joint, where at an angle of 95°, tension within fibers is highest or strength mobilization is greatest. Said another way, range of motion provides a basis for suboptimal and optimal crossbridge interaction. (Courtesy of Elizabeth A. Drum)

Force–Velocity Relationship

In accordance with the length–tension discussion, force–velocity variables also change the dynamics of skeletal muscle interaction. Simply stated, the force–velocity relationship indicates that as the speed of a muscular action increases, force production drops and vice versa [10]. This can be important during the rehabilitation of a patient or performance training of a client to insure that force development is optimized for whatever the outcome goal might be. For instance, to maximize force production in skeletal muscle, slower and controlled movement is probably warranted to optimize progressive overload manifested as greater force development in the musculature. On the other hand, if the goal is to improve speed or endurance, then it might be necessary to add a speed component to the performance of muscular actions along with understanding that force in the form of resistance needs to decline. In other words, the force–velocity relationship should guide training and rehabilitation to reflect that sport-specific or even every-day life activities are not slow and controlled but rather quick and sometimes unanticipated. Figure 2.3 showcases the force–velocity relationship.

Motor Innervation

Neuromotor System Arrangement

Recall that to initiate the SFT, sufficient neuromotor stimulus had to be realized. Let us look at this in a bit more detail but still from a big picture perspective. Most efferent ("output") electrical signals begin with central nervous system (CNS) involvement and end with peripheral nervous system (PNS) activation, while afferent ("input") signals relay sensory information from peripheral areas to the spinal cord and CNS. Recall, then, that the human nervous system is made up of primarily the CNS (i.e., brain and spinal cord) and PNS (i.e., nerves that transmit electrical waves to and from the CNS) [5]. In relation to skeletal muscle physiology, CNS and PNS input both travel to the muscle fiber to influence muscular

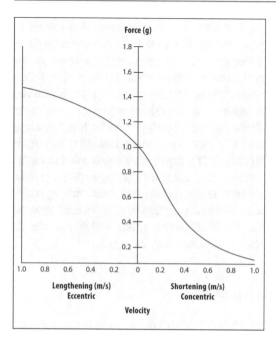

Fig. 2.3 The force–velocity relationship of muscle action. During eccentric action, as the speed of fiber lengthening under tension increases, so does muscle tension. The opposite is true during concentric action or shortening of the fiber under tension whereby tension decreases as the speed of fiber shortening increases. (Courtesy of Elizabeth A. Drum)

action at the neuromuscular junction effecting the action potential (AP) and motor unit properties.

The SFT—Action Potential (AP) and Muscle Fiber Motor Unit Integration

The primary mechanism, physically responsible for force production, in the SFT is the filaments themselves. This process of sliding filaments is primarily regulated by afferent and efferent neurological signals via APs, where sodium (Na^+) and potassium (K^+) are exchanged across neuronal and muscle cell membranes. Eventually, the AP is propagated deep inside a muscle fiber, via transverse tubules (T-tubules), and triggers Ca^{2+} release from the sarcoplasmic reticulum (SR) into the sarcoplasm. Ca^{2+} then binds with troponin, a protein on actin. Suddenly troponin, through a conformational change, pulls another protein, tropomyosin—a long, winding, and thin

stranded structure—off actin's active sites. Myosin's energized heads interact with actin and excitation–contraction coupling ensues [10]. What follows are definitions and phases of muscle action related to the SFT—with all its moving parts in a regulated and force-producing sequence.

Constituent Structures of the SFT

Myofibrils

Each muscle fiber contains several hundred to several thousand myofibrils. Myofibrils are arranged in a three-dimensional mosaic pattern and contain the basic contractile structures or proteins—actin and myosin (also known as thin and thick filaments, respectively, a common theme we identified prior)—of a muscle fiber. Additionally, recall that the smallest contractile unit of a muscle fiber is termed the sarcomere which is made up of thin and thick filaments.

Microscopically, a distinctive striped or striated appearance is observed when viewing myofibrils. These striations are apparent due to the thin and thick structural appearance of muscle. The mid-portion of a sarcomere that appears to be dark is known as the A-band and is formed because both thick and thin filaments overlap in this region. The lighter areas on the outer ends are known as I-bands. The lighter appearance occurs because only thin filaments are located in this range. The H-zone is located within the central region of the A-band, where no thick and thin filament overlap is evident. A dark line in the middle of the H-zone is termed the M-line. The M-line is composed of proteins that help aid the sarcomere in maintaining spatial orientation as the fiber lengthens and shortens (i.e., relaxes and contracts, respectively). The I-band is interrupted by a dark stripe, another protein structure, referred to as the Z-disk or Z-line, which serves as an anchor or attachment point for actin.

As the sarcomere is the basic fundamental contractile unit of a muscle cell, each cell is composed of a plethora of sarcomeres joined end to end. To summarize, each sarcomere contains the following aforementioned regions: I-bands (light zone), A-band (dark zone), H-zone, and M-line. Furthermore, sarcomeres are joined together at the Z-disks with the help of two proteins, titin and nebulin, which help provide points of attachment and stability for thin filaments. Interestingly, titin is now considered a possible third filament, serving as a "spring-like" attachment to the Z-line along with actin [12]. Following are more detailed descriptions of the individual types of myofilaments.

Thick Filament (Myosin)

The principal protein of the thick filament is myosin. Myosin accounts for nearly one half to two thirds of the total myofibrillar protein. Each myosin filament is typically formed by 200 or more myosin molecules. Myosin is a hexameric molecule consisting of one pair of myosin heavy chains and two pairs of light chains. These proteins twist together with one end forming a globular head, called the myosin head. Within each thick filament, many myosin heads are formed and protrude to form crossbridges that interact with specialized activation sites on the thin filament during muscular contraction. An array of fine filaments composed of titin extend from Z-disk to M-line that aid in stabilizing the myosin filaments along the longitudinal axis [10].

Thin Filament

Each thin filament is composed of three different proteins—actin, tropomyosin, and troponin. However, thin filament is often referred to simply as an actin filament. Thin filament has one end inserted into the Z-disk with the aid of nebulin anchoring the filament in place and the opposite end extending to the center of the sarcomere. Also, keep in mind that titin also interacts with actin and quite possibly helps anchor it to the Z-line [12]. Furthermore, thin filament is located in the space between thick filaments [5].

Individual actin molecules are globular proteins (known as G-actin) that join together to form the backbone of thin filaments. Two strands of actin-derived filaments twist in a helical pattern. Twisting around the actin strands is a tube-shaped protein called tropomyosin. Yet another protein, a more complex protein called troponin, is attached at regular intervals to both actin and tropomyosin. Troponin and tropomyosin work together along with Ca^{2+} ions to maintain relaxation or initiate an action of the myofibril. Keep in mind that actin and myosin work in unison to help promote muscle movement, such as an isotonic action, which is the cornerstone of how you do "work" (remember $W = F \times D$) when lifting weights or simply walking, among many other tasks.

Sarcoplasm

Within the plasma membrane is the sarcoplasm, a muscle fiber's cytoplasm. This area is rich in soluble proteins, minerals, high-energy intermediates, substrates, enzymes of metabolism, mitochondrial protein, and other necessary organelles. Additionally, Ca^{2+} flux will occur into and out of this medium as part of the SFT. The sarcoplasm differs from cytoplasm of other cells due to the high quantity of stored glycogen as well as myoglobin, an oxygen-binding compound (or protein) similar to hemoglobin [5, 10].

Transverse Tubules (T-tubules)

T-tubules are an extensive network of extensions of the plasma membrane that pass laterally through and deep into the muscle fiber. Due to the interconnected pathways of these tubules through the myofibrils, APs can be rapidly transmitted to individual myofibrils from superficial to deep. The tubules also act as a pathway for external substances to enter the cell and waste products to leave the interior of the muscle fiber. Each T-tubule lies between two enlarged portions of the SR called cisternae. These three structures (SR, T-tubules, and cisternae) form a triad near the region where actin and myosin overlap [10].

Sarcoplasmic Reticulum (SR)

The SR, which corresponds to the endoplasmic reticulum of other cells, is a longitudinal network of tubules that parallel myofibrils and wrap around them. The SR is a storage site for Ca^{2+} which is a critical component for muscular contraction as introduced above [5].

Along with depolarizing the muscle fiber membrane, the AP travels over the T-tubule network and directly into the fiber toward the SR. The SR has a high concentration of Ca^{2+} ions compared to the sarcoplasm due to an active (i.e., ATP requiring) calcium pump in the SR membrane. In response to the muscle impulse (i.e., AP), the SR cisternae or terminal sacs housing Ca^{2+} become more permeable and the Ca^{2+} ions diffuse into the sarcoplasm.

Phases of the SFT—The Big Picture of Microscopic Muscle Action

Muscle Fiber Resting Phase

During resting conditions, most Ca^{2+} is stored in the SR, so little Ca^{2+} is in the myofibril. Therefore, very few myosin crossbridges are attached to actin and little to no tension is maintained in the musculature. Hence, at this time the muscle is considered to be in a resting state with actin's active sites covered by tropomyosin.

Excitation Coupling Phase

Subsequently, when Ca^{2+} ions are released from the SR into the sarcoplasm, they bind to troponin on actin filaments, effectively changing the conformation of troponin. Troponin, therefore, initiates the contraction process by moving tropomyosin strands, through a chemical, conformational change, from the myosin-binding sites on actin. The fiber's contractile proteins have now gone from a resting state to an active state. Furthermore, once tropomyosin has been shifted off of actin's binding sites (i.e., myosin-binding sites),

the myosin heads are able to attach, allowing crossbridge (i.e., the attachment of the myosin head to actin's active site) flexion to occur [13]. The force produced at any time is directly related to the number of myosin crossbridge heads bound to actin filaments at that instant [14]. This might explain genetic differences in strength potential or development and, therefore, variances in sport performance based on variable training adaptations. Conversely, keep in mind that a loss of muscle fibers, such as during deconditioning, injury, or aging, is associated with a loss of force production and, therefore, inadequate myosin crossbridge formation, among other degradations.

Recall that every muscle fiber is functionally connected to an axon of a motor neuron. Specifically, an α motor neuron connects and innervates many muscle fibers. Notably, as mentioned previously, a motor unit is an α motor neuron and all the muscle fibers it innervates. The site of functional connection, not physical connection, occurs at the synapse.

To review, in order for a muscular action to occur, an AP or electrical signal must be initiated from the brain or spinal cord to an α motor neuron. The AP arrives at the dendrites of the α motor neuron and eventually travels down the axon to the axon terminal. After the AP reaches the axon terminal, acetylcholine (ACh) secretion is initiated. ACh is a neurotransmitter synthesized in the cytoplasm of the motor neuron and in the distal end of the axon. ACh is then released into the synaptic cleft and binds to specific receptors in the muscle fiber membrane (on the postsynaptic membrane). This causes an increase in the permeability of Na^+ ions and stimulates a muscle impulse due to the entry of these charged particles into the muscle fiber. This process is known as depolarization. Repolarization occurs when K^+ effluxes from inside to outside a cell, such as with a fiber or dendrite. Na^+/K^+ membrane potentials are maintained, then, via the Na^+/K^+ ATPase pumps, which continuously facilitate active transport of the aforementioned ions across the muscle membrane to maintain a polarized state.

Contraction Phase

With the above protein interactions in mind, recall that there needs to be a sufficient amount of energy available in the form of ATP for muscular action to occur and/or be maintained. For crossbridge flexion or action, energy is derived from the hydrolysis of ATP to ADP and P_i. This reaction is catalyzed by the enzyme myosin adenosine triphosphatase (ATPase) in the myosin head, where energy release is captured and held until "contraction" or crossbridge shortening occurs. After "contraction," an ATP molecule must replace the ADP molecule on the myosin crossbridge or head in order for the myosin head to detach from the actin site and be able to re-cock (and to attach again as needed). Thus, during the muscle action, the ADP structure detaches so that ATP is able to bind to the myosin head. Next, the myosin head detaches from actin and falls back into a re-cocked position. Spontaneously the ATP molecule is then enzymatically split to ADP + P_i + energy, whereby the energy is "held" in the myosin head. Now the energized crossbridge or myosin head is ready to attach to actin's active sites and pull actin toward the center of the sarcomere as needed. This causes a muscular contraction (or action) by creating greater overlap of the actin and myosin filaments and decreasing the length of the sarcomere. This process continues as long as ATP is present, nerve impulses release ACh, and enough Ca^{2+} is available in the sarcoplasm to bind to troponin; otherwise, relaxation occurs and very few crossbridges remain. Collectively this cyclical process is termed excitation–contraction coupling [15].

Relaxation Phase

As suggested prior, relaxation in the muscle fiber occurs primarily when nerve impulses cease to exist and Ca^{2+} is actively taken up into the SR. Thus, there are a few main events that occur during relaxation. First, the remaining ACh in the synapse is rapidly broken down by acetylcholinesterase. This enzyme prevents the continuous stimulation of a muscle fiber from a nerve impulse. Second, ACh is no longer a stimulus for the sarcolemma. Moreover, active Ca^{2+} pumps rapidly move Ca^{2+} back into the SR, causing greater Ca^{2+} concentrations in the SR than the sarcoplasm. As the myosin crossbridge links break, tropomyosin again covers actin's active sites, effectually blocking and preventing crossbridge attachment. It is important to note that ATP is required for *relaxation* to occur. At this point, the muscle fiber remains relaxed and energized awaiting the opening of actin's active site (i.e., from an appropriate nerve impulse and Ca^{2+} release into the sarcoplasm). Figure 2.4 succinctly summarizes the SFT.

Proprioceptors in Muscles, Joints, and Tendons

Last but not least, let us explore a brief flurry of information derived from the musculoskeletal system itself. These proprioceptors provide information to protect or enhance a muscular action and our awareness of limb movement. In short, muscles spindles, Golgi tendon organs (GTO), and Pacinian corpuscles are the main receptor we will discuss. They all serve to enhance our ability to move or mobilize muscle in a coordinated and protected fashion. "Proprioception can be defined as the cumulative neural input to the central nervous system from specialized nerve endings called mechanoreceptors," according to Ribeiro et al. [16].

With that in mind, let us discuss the primary proprioceptor, muscle spindles, which provide mechanosensory feedback regarding alterations in skeletal muscle fiber length and tension [5]. Foremost, the spindles, which are wrapped around intrafusal fibers surrounded by extrafusal fibers, provide feedback about muscle stretch and, therefore, will initiate a counteraction if too much stretch is "sensed." This opposing action is in the form of a contraction whereby the muscle belly shortens, avoiding a potential "over-stretch" of the fiber. Interestingly, this might be advantageous to power development (e.g., plyometric-type exercise) in that a greater force-producing effort may be realized if the "stretch reflex" is

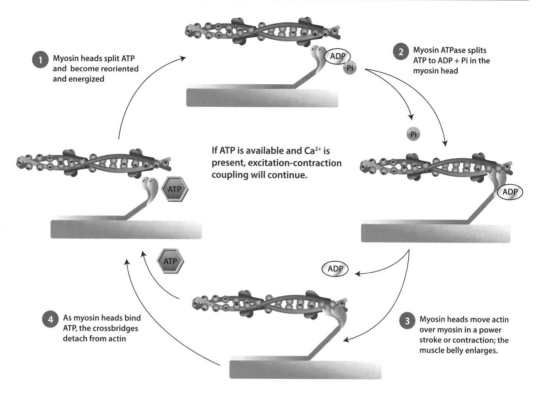

1. Myosin heads split ATP and become reoriented and energized

2. Myosin ATPase splits ATP to ADP + Pi in the myosin head

If ATP is available and Ca²⁺ is present, excitation-contraction coupling will continue.

4. As myosin heads bind ATP, the crossbridges detach from actin

3. Myosin heads move actin over myosin in a power stroke or contraction; the muscle belly enlarges.

Fig. 2.4 Microscopic view of the sliding filament theory (SFT) in a single fiber. Note that ATP is the primary driver of this process. When ATP binds to the myosin head, crossbridge dissociation occurs and ATP is split to ADP + Pi + energy captured in the myosin head until the head reattaches to actin and a power stroke is realized. Thus, metabolic production of ATP is the ultimate driver of sustained muscle action. (Courtesy of Elizabeth A. Drum)

invoked. In short, this is due to a stretch-shortening cycle (SSC) [17] phenomenon whereby the series elastic component of muscle (i.e., tendons) stores energy and along with stretch reflex activation, maximal enhancement of muscle recruitment over a short time period is realized. Furthermore, the parallel elastic component (i.e., epimysium, perimysium, endomysium, and sarcolemma; discussed in Chap. 3) of muscle reacts with a passive force [17]. Collectively, the SSC and muscle spindle activation helps the relay of information related to dynamic movement and interaction with conscious and subconscious areas of the CNS. Importantly, proprioception is largely outside of conscious control most of the time, contributing to functions such as maintaining posture or position of body parts [17]. Moreover, it is efficient not to "think" about our body in space during every day activities and to react reflexively during sport performance.

Another proprioceptive entity is the GTO. This sensor is located in tendons near the myotendinous junction. It is positioned in series or end to end in extrafusal muscle fibers. When activated by a *significantly* large load on the muscle, the GTO sends afferent signals to an interneuron in the spinal cord that synapses with and inhibits a motor neuron aligning with the same muscle [17]. You may have predicted that the end result of this feedback is a decline in tension on the muscle and tendon. Thus, GTOs cause the muscle to inactivate versus muscle spindles that cause muscle to react or activate (i.e., shorten). Taken together, both types of proprioceptors serve a protective function and relay information to the nervous system about potential changes in body movement that could be harmful. On the other hand, both spindles and GTOs may assist with exercise or sport performance by helping with increased force production. Recall that muscle spindles are part of the SSC occurrence. As for GTOs, resistance training may modify GTO activation by training the motor cortex to override GTO inhibitory effects and thereby allow for greater force realization in an overloaded muscle [17].

The third and final mechanoreceptor to be discussed is the Pacinian corpuscle. This structure is found in tendon sheaths and intramuscular connective tissue. Generally, it is thought of as a large and highly structured end organ in cutaneous and tendinous tissue and is predominantly susceptible to high-velocity changes in limb acceleration and deceleration [18]. Therefore, the Pacinian corpuscle quickly adjusts at the start of joint movements during rapid changes in stress.

For example, closed chain movements may be especially suitable for rapid joint movements at a variety of velocities. This could modify the Pacinian corpuscles [18], among other mechanoreceptors.

Finally, a vital point is that proprioception tends to decline with age and is compounded by a lack of consistent and deliberate physical activity. For the most part, the muscle spindles tend to become less effective than the GTOs over time. Keeping in mind that proprioception is a combination of joint position sense and the sense of limb movement, both of which are important components of producing a smooth and coordinated joint movement [16]. The significance of

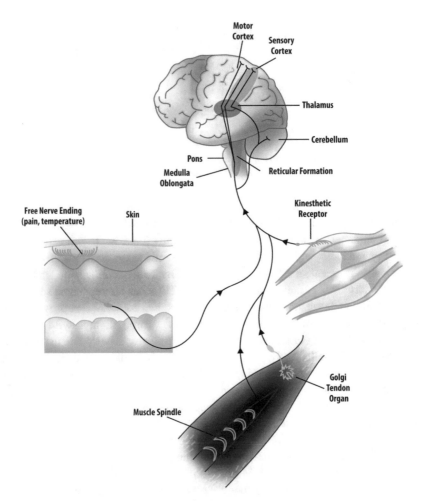

Fig. 2.5 The interaction of a muscle spindle and *Golgi tendon organ* (GTO) in relation to muscle action. The spindles cause the muscle to "contract" when too much stretch is sensed and the GTOs respond by causing the muscle to "relax" if too much tension is realized. (Courtesy of Elizabeth A. Drum)

this is that if a person progressively becomes less functional in their ability to detect a joint angle or passive motion of a limb, they become more likely to lose balance and fall. Therefore, consistent exercise tends to positively modulate morphological characteristics in mechanoreceptors, namely the primary sensor or muscle spindles, as we age [16]. Ultimately, by maintaining large muscle movement activity, such as walking, running, and/or resistance training throughout the lifespan, proprioception at both the peripheral and central levels is maintained or improved. Figure 2.5 illustrates the key proprioceptors discussed prior.

Acknowledgment The authors warmly thank Elizabeth A. Drum for her time, efforts, and expertly drawn figures.

References

1. Bergstrom J, Hermansen L, Hultman E, et al. Diet, muscle glycogen and physical performance. Acta Physiol Scand. 1967;71:140–50.
2. Foskett A, Williams C, Boobis L, et al. Carbohydrate availability and muscle energy metabolism during intermittent running. Med Sci Sports Exerc. 2008;40:96–103.
3. Green HJ, Ball-Burnett M, Jones S, et al. Mechanical and metabolic responses with exercise and dietary carbohydrate manipulation. Med Sci Sports Exerc. 2007;39:139–48.
4. Murakami I, Sakuragi T, Uemura H, et al. Significant effect of a pre-exercise high-fat meal after a 3-day high-carbohydrate diet on endurance performance. Nutrients. 2012;4:625–37.
5. McArdle WD, Katch FI, Katch VL. Exercise physiology: nutrition, energy, and human performance. 7th ed. Philadelphia: Wolters Kluwer; 2010.
6. Enoka RM. Morphological features and activation patterns of motor units. J Clin Neurophysiol. 1995;12:538–59.
7. Huxley H, Hanson J. Changes in the cross-striations of muscle during contraction and stretch and their structural interpretation. Nature. 1954;173:973–6.
8. Huxley A, Niedergerke R. Structural changes in muscle during contraction: interference microscopy of living muscle fibres. Nature. 1954;173:971–3.
9. Huxley A. Muscle structure and theories of contraction. Prog Biophys Biophys Chem. 1957;7:255–318.
10. Brooks GA, Fahey TD, Baldwin KM. Exercise physiology: human bioenergetics and its applications. 4th ed. Boston: McGraw-Hill; 2005.
11. Rassier D, MacIntosh BR, Herzog W. Length dependence of active force production in skeletal muscle. J Appl Physiol. 1999;86:1445–57.
12. Farrell PA, Joyner MJ, Caiozzo VJ, et al. ACSM's advanced exercise physiology. 2nd ed. Philadelphia: Wolters Kluwer Health; 2012.
13. Komi PV, IOC Medical Commission, International Federation of Sports Medicine. Strength and power in sport. 2nd ed. Osney Mead: Blackwell; 2003.
14. Stone M, O'bryant H. Weight training: a scientific approach. 2nd ed. Minneapolis: Burgess; 1987.
15. Sandow A. Excitation-contraction coupling in muscular response. Yale J Biol Med. 1952;25:176–201.
16. Ribeiro F, Oliveira, J. Aging effects on joint proprioception: the role of physical activity in proprioception preservation. Eur Rev Aging Phys Act. 2007;4:71–6.
17. Baechle TR, Earle RW, National Strength & Conditioning Association (U.S.). Essentials of strength training and conditioning. 3rd ed. Champaign: Human Kinetics; 2008.
18. Bunton EE, Pitney, William A, Cappaert, Thomas A, Kane, Alexander W. The role of limb torque, muscle action and proprioception during closed kinetic chain rehabilitation of the lower extremity. J Athl Train. 1993;28:10–11, 14, 16, 19–[20].

Structure and Organization of Skeletal Muscle

3

J. Bryan Dixon, Scott N. Drum and Ryan Weatherwax

Introduction

Skeletal muscle can be studied and understood at a variety of scales or levels. Recall that Chap. 1 considered the gross anatomy of the leg. This classical approach to anatomy informs many of our clinical assumptions and discussions. However, a reliance on gross anatomy can be misleading or less informative. For instance, fascial connections can beguile attempts to isolate muscle function, while the size and shape of muscles can lead to faulty inferences about in vivo muscle function. Chapter 2 focused on the molecular structure of skeletal muscle. This molecular and cellular approach provides the basis to understanding the physiological principles of skeletal muscle. However, understanding muscle function on a physiological scale provides an incomplete explanation of the variability seen in clinical muscle function or human performance.

Therefore, this chapter will focus on an intermediate scale, where we discuss the internal structure of skeletal muscle, a bridge between gross anatomy and molecular physiology. We begin with a general and idealized description of skeletal muscle architecture before moving to a more detailed discussion. Skeletal muscle architecture reveals surprising insights into the functional properties of individual muscles and has important clinical corollaries. Skeletal muscle architecture, or "design," can be viewed as a hierarchical matrix. In this perspective, the individual constituent components are arranged to form a composite structure that gives rise to many of the properties that we recognize at the clinical level as individual muscle function. The chapter concludes with a discussion of skeletal muscle connective tissue and satellite cells.

General Muscle Architecture Categories

Muscle fibers, also known as muscle cells, are elongated and cylindrical in shape. They have varying and mutable diameters, which at largest approximate the average diameter of a human hair. Muscle fiber length is also highly variable with the longest fibers of the sartorius muscle reaching 40 cm in length. The number of muscle fibers within a single muscle range from several hundred to more than a million. The internal architecture of a muscle is largely determined by the characteristics and arrangement of these muscle fibers. Furthermore, patterns of muscle fiber arrangements produce morphological features of muscles that have given

J. B. Dixon (✉)
Sports Medicine, Advanced Center for Orthopedics, Marquette, MI, USA
e-mail: jbryandixon@hotmail.com

S. N. Drum
School of Health and Human Performance, Northern Michigan University, Marquette, MI, USA
e-mail: sdrum@nmu.edu

R. Weatherwax
Department of Recreation and Exercise and Sports Science, Western State Colorado University, Gunnison, CO, USA

rise to a commonly used muscle classification schema designating muscles as parallel or pennate.

Parallel muscles are defined by the relatively parallel arrangement of muscle fibers to the axis of pull of the tendon. Parallel muscles are often further classified as flat or fusiform. Fusiform muscles are thicker in the middle and taper toward the ends (i.e., biceps brachii). This spindle shape is often used for the classic illustration of an idealized muscle.

Pennate muscles derive their name from the Latin *penna* for feather and share many analogous features of vaned feathers. In a vaned feather, branches or barbs attach at an angle to a central shaft or rachis, while in a pennate muscle, the muscle fibers attach at an angle to a tendon. The degree of obliquity of the fiber relative to the axis of pull of the tendon is the defining feature of pennate muscles and is described by the pennation angle. This architectural arrangement results in reduced force acting along the axis of pull of the tendon per fiber, but allows for more fibers to be packed into the muscle resulting in an overall increase in force production compared to a muscle of parallel design with a similar anatomical cross-sectional area. Pennate muscles are further classified as unipennate, bipennate, or multipennate.

Although commonly used to describe individual skeletal muscles, these general categories are the idealized schemas. Describing a muscle as parallel or pennate does not capture the complexity of muscle fiber arrangements in vivo. Nevertheless, looking at the extremes of parallel and multipennate architecture provides important insight into the importance of the architectural structure of muscle and the impact on function.

Anatomical and Physiologic Cross-Sectional Area

The greater the pennation angle and the more complex the pennation pattern, the more muscle fibers can be packed into a muscle and the greater force it can generate. Because of the effect of pennation angle and pattern on force production, the physiological cross-sectional area (PSCA) is a more accurate assessment of force potential than anatomical cross-sectional area. This

is one example where relying on gross anatomy can lead to less predictive assumptions about the potential for muscle force development. While anatomical cross-sectional area corresponds relatively well to force generation in muscles with parallel architecture, using anatomical cross section underestimates the force generation of pennate muscles as it fails to account for the oblique and shorter fibers that do not span the thickest part of the muscle, but contribute equally to force generation. As described below, PSCA, measured perpendicular to the muscle fibers, helps solve this problem and is a more accurate way to assess force potential of a given muscle.

As discussed in Chap. 2, skeletal muscle is composed of slow- and fast-twitch fiber variations. These fiber types convey different functional properties. At the extremes of fiber types and performance demands, the effect or influence of fiber type is glaringly apparent (e.g., slow-twitch marathoner vs. a fast-twitch sprinter). However, it should be noted that during routine performance demands for the general population the effect of fiber type is modest. The effect size of fiber type on muscle performance is further reduced by adaptations that occur during dedicated training programs. This is not to dismiss the importance of muscle fiber type in the physiology of skeletal muscle, but rather to caution against the tendency to overemphasize the importance of fiber type at the expense of other considerations of skeletal muscle function; a tendency which may stem from the familiarly with fiber type differences and the ease of measuring fiber type for both research and performance purposes.

Emergent Properties of the Sarcomere

As discussed in Chap. 2, muscle fiber contraction is a complex process that involves cellular and chemical interactions. Recall that the smallest contractile unit of a muscle is termed the sarcomere, which is made up of thin (actin) and thick (myosin) filaments. Sarcomeres are joined end to end at the Z-disk or Z-line to create a myofibril. Hundreds to thousands of myofibrils are bundled together to form the cellular contractile unit of a muscle fiber.

The variability in myofibril length, known as serial sarcomere number, determines the distance a muscle fiber can shorten. The number of myofibrils within a muscle fiber, known as parallel sarcomere number, determines the potential force of the muscle fiber. The contractile properties of a sarcomere are functionally equivalent in all human skeletal muscles. Each sarcomere can generate an equivalent force and shorten an equivalent distance. Therefore, the number of sarcomeres arranged in series determines the distance a muscle fiber can shorten (often referred to as the muscle's excursion) and the number of sarcomeres arranged in parallel determines the force capability of an individual muscle fiber.

A muscle fiber with long myofibrils has a high excursion potential. A muscle fiber that packs in many myofibrils will have high force potential. These two architectural properties of the muscle fiber, myofibril length and myofibril density, determine the excursion and force potential of an individual muscle fiber. The functional properties of an individual muscle have been shown to correlate closely with the sum of these muscle fiber properties within that muscle. Therefore, to understand the properties of an individual muscle at the clinical level requires an understanding of the characteristics of the individual muscle fibers within that muscle.

Myofibril density is approximated using the PSCA of the muscle. This value is calculated using the mass of the muscle (m), the fiber length of the muscle (L), the pennation angle $(cos\theta)$, and a constant for muscle density (ρ) [1].

$$PSCA = m \cdot \cos\theta \, / \rho \cdot L$$

Because muscle fiber length usually correlates closely with myofibril length, muscle fiber length is used as a marker for excursion potential or velocity. Therefore, muscle fiber length is used to determine excursion, while PSCA is used to determine force. The force–velocity relationship inherent in internal muscle design indicates that as the speed of a muscular action increases, force production drops and vice versa.

Based on these relationships, we can predict that there will be inherent trade-offs in muscle function based on the particular design of a muscle. If a muscle has both long fibers and a large cross-sectional area, it will be capable of both high excursion and high force, but will necessarily have a high mass and metabolic demand. On the other hand, muscles with long fibers, but small cross-sectional area, will have high excursion but low force potential. Contrary to the prior statement, muscles with a large cross-sectional area, but short fibers will have high force and low excursion potential. A fourth possibility would be observing short fibers with a small cross-sectional area. These muscles would have low mass and metabolic demand, but limited force and movement potential.

With the inherent trade-offs in function, we would expect muscles to be specialized to their functional role, so only the necessary features to accomplish the range of performance required would be present. That is, we would expect the structure of muscle to closely follow from the function of that muscle. Dr. Sam Ward has developed this concept of structural–functional relationships for muscles of the lower extremity by experientially determining the structure of individual muscles and proposing general categories for these specialized functions. Table 3.1 shows the experimentally determined architectural values for muscles of the leg.

The data obtained by Ward suggest that muscles tend to fall into particular categories of architectural design and, hence, categories of function. Ward has developed functional categories based on these data that have particular practical relevance for clinicians and performance specialists. Stabilizing muscles, which exhibit high force potential, have a large PSCA, and small fiber length. Mobility muscles, which have a high excursion potential, are made up of long fibers but small cross-sectional area. Super muscles have both long fibers and high cross-sectional areas. Joint tuning muscles have small fiber length and small cross-sectional area. These data-driven schemas are helpful in understanding the functional specialization of individual muscles and have particular practical relevance for clinicians and performance specialists. Table 3.2 and Fig. 3.1.

Table 3.1 Architectural properties of leg muscles. (Adapted from: [2]. With permission from Springer Publishing)

Muscle	Mass (g)	Muscle length (cm)	Fiber length (cm)	Lf coefficient of variation (%)	Ls (μm)	Pennation angle (°)	PCSA (cm²)	Lf/Lm ratio
Tibialis anterior ($n=21$)	80.1±26.6	25.98±3.25	6.83±0.79	6.6±4.0	3.14±0.16	9.6±3.1	10.9±3.0	0.27±0.05
Extensor hallucis longus ($n=21$)	20.9±9.9	24.25±3.27	7.48±1.13	7.7±5.7	3.24±0.11	9.4±2.2	2.7±1.5	0.31±0.06
Extensor digitorum longus ($n=21$)	41.0±12.6	29.00±2.33	6.93±1.14	8.0±4.4	3.12±0.20	10.8±2.8	5.6±1.7	0.24±0.04
Peroneus longus ($n=19$)	57.7±22.6	27.08±3.02	5.08±0.63	10.4±6.5	2.72±0.25	14.1±5.1	10.4±3.8	0.19±0.03
Peroneus brevis ($n=20$)	24.2±10.6	23.75±3.11	4.54±0.65	10.1±6.0	2.76±0.19	11.5±3.0	4.9±2.0	0.19±0.03
Gastrocnemius medial head ($n=20$)	113.5±32.0	26.94±4.65	5.10±0.98	13.4±7.0	2.59±0.26	9.9±4.4	21.1±5.7	0.19±0.03
Gastrocnemius lateral head ($n=20$)	62.2±24.6	22.35±3.70	5.88±0.95	15.8±11.2	2.71±0.24	12.0±3.1	9.7±3.3	0.27±0.03
Soleus ($n=19$)	275.8±98.5	40.54±8.32	4.40±0.99	16.7±6.9	2.12±0.24	28.3±10.1	51.8±14.9	0.11±0.02
Flexor hallucis longus ($n=19$)	38.9±17.1	26.88±3.55	5.27±1.29	9.7±5.7	2.37±0.24	16.9±4.6	6.9±2.7	0.20±0.05
Flexor digitorum longus ($n=19$)	20.3±10.8	27.33±5.62	4.46±1.06	9.6±5.0	2.56±0.25	13.6±4.7	4.4±2.0	0.16±0.09
Tibialis posterior ($n=20$)	58.4±19.2	31.03±4.68	3.78±0.49	9.1±5.6	2.56±0.32	13.7±4.1	14.4±4.9	0.12±0.02

Values are expressed as mean ± standard deviation

Lf fiber length normalized to a sarcomere length of 2.7 μm, Ls sarcomere length, Lm muscle length normalized to a sarcomere length of 2.7 μm; PSCA physiologic cross-sectional area

Table 3.2 Summary of the structure function trade-offs in skeletal muscle design

	Long fiber length	Short fiber length
Large cross-sectional area	Super muscles (high dynamic force)	Stabilizer muscles (high static force)
Small cross-sectional area	Mobility muscles (high excursion/velocity)	Joint tuning muscles (low static and dynamic force)

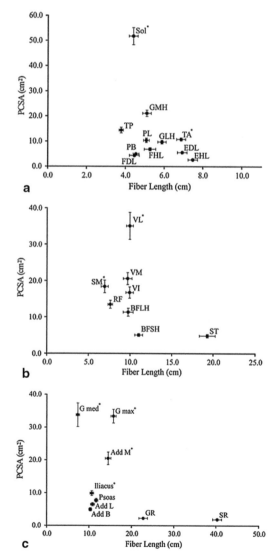

Fig. 3.1 Scatterplots of muscle *fiber length* versus *PCSA* for the **a** ankle, **b** knee, and **c** hip are shown. **a** At the ankle, the muscles follow the classic trade-off between *PCSA* and *fiber length*; large *PCSA* correlates with short fibers. Also at the ankle, plantarflexor and dorsiflexor fiber lengths are dramatically different from those of

Furthermore, when muscles are analyzed as a functional group, the associated muscles often have unique structural designs and, therefore, different functional specializations. These combinations appear to be synergistic, allowing for a broad range of function with maximal efficiency. As an example of this phenomenon, Leiber observed that in the upper extremity synergetic muscles with unique design properties allowed for reduced total mass (as much as 30%) compared to the requirements for a single muscle to meet an equivalent performance spectrum [1].

Length–Tension Relationship Inherent in Internal Muscle Design

The length of a muscle fiber relative to its optimal length is critical in determining the amount of force or tension that can be developed. The optimal length can be defined as the length of the sarcomere, or the smallest contractile unit of a fiber, that provides ideal overlap of thick and thin filaments. Therefore, when optimal length is obtained in a sarcomere, the greatest amount of force production is possible because of optimal

previous reports. **b** At the knee, the quadriceps and hamstrings have opposite architectural trends. The quadriceps muscles range from short-fibered, small *PCSA* to long-fibered, large *PCSA*, whereas the hamstrings follow the classic pattern of short fibers, large *PCSA* to long fibers, and small *PCSA*. Importantly, the vastus lateralis would be expected to dominate function. **c** At the hip, the muscles follow the classic trade-off between *fiber length* and *PCSA*. The gluteus medius and maximus would be expected to dominate function. *PCSA* physiologic cross-sectional area, *Sol* soleus, *GMH* gastrocnemius medial head, *LMH* gastrocnemius lateral head, *TP* tibialis posterior, *PL* peroneus longus, *PB* peroneus brevis, *FHL* flexor hallucis longus, *FDL* flexor digitorum longus, *TA* tibialis anterior, *EHL* extensor hallucis longus, *EDL* extensor digitorum longus, *VL* vastus lateralis, *VM* vastus medialis, *VI* vastus intermedius, *RF* rectus femoris, *ST* semitendinosus, *SM* semimembranosus, *BFLH* biceps femoris lateral head, *BFSH* biceps femoris short head, *G med* gluteus medius, *G max* gluteus maximus, *Add M* adductor magnus, *Add L* adductor longus, *Add B* adductor brevis, *GR* gracilis, *SR* sartorius. All values are plotted as mean ± standard error. *=muscles with the largest ($p<0.05$) PCSA in their respective muscle group. (From: [2]. Reprinted with permission from Springer Publishing) actin–myosin interaction. Increases or decreases beyond this optimal level (either shorter or longer) result in reduced force potential. Hence, when a muscle is shorter or longer than optimal length, there is impairment in maximal or optimal force production. This suggests that muscles are also designed to operate within a relatively narrow range of length. Changes in muscle length, both due to natural or iatrogenic causes, will likely change the functional properties of the muscle, and may have a concomitant effect on the broader functional muscle groups related to that muscle. Therefore, determining and attempting to restore optimal length is critical in surgical and rehabilitation efforts [3].

One caveat to the length sensitive nature of muscles in force production occurs during eccentric action. Eccentric actions result in a net increase of energy into the muscle and cause the cross bridges to attach stronger. This leads to the somewhat counterintuitive fact that muscles can resist more force than they are capable of generating. Some muscles appear to have specific design features that are specialized to store the passive energy of eccentric actions resulting in functional advantages. Therefore, understanding the passive properties of individual muscles and the associated soft tissue is also important in understanding function.

Passive Properties of Muscles and Connective Tissue in Skeletal Muscle Design

Fascia, considered as a dense connective tissue, holds a muscle in place and provides separation from adjacent muscles and structures. Fascia extends beyond the ends of muscle fibers to form slings of connective tissue and cordlike tendons. The tendon serves as an anchor by intertwining with the periosteum, or outer layer, of bone. Additionally, the associated fascia form fibrous sheets called aponeuroses, which allow for the interaction of the muscle with bone or outer layers of adjacent muscles. In actuality, fascia layers give the entire muscular system "flexibility" to move around within a defined but fluid space [4].

Fascia also plays a role in chronic injuries and can contribute to clinically relevant problems, such as chronic exertional compartment syndrome. Chronic exertional compartment syndrome is manifested by symptomatically elevated intracompartmental pressure within inelastic fascia and is particularly common in the lower extremities [5]. All in all, when considering the structure of skeletal muscle, be aware of multiple layers of connective tissue and the role fascia can play in injury and functional limitations.

Taking a closer look at fascia of skeletal muscle, you will see three distinct fascia layers viewed from superficial to deep. The entire outside circumference of skeletal muscle is surrounded by the epimysium (from the Greek prefix epi—above or upon and suffix mysium—abstract noun for muscle) just beneath the skin, which allows for free movement of skin. Next, deeper versus the former layer, bundles of muscle fibers exist called fascicles that are enveloped by the perimysium (near or encircling the muscle), which surrounds each fascicle containing many muscle fibers. Around each individual muscle fiber is the endomysium (inside or within the muscle). The function of the endomysium and perimysium remains under investigation, but likely contribute, along with titin and other muscle cell structures, to unique passive mechanical tension properties of particular muscles. Figure 3.2 depicts the various fascia layers.

The endomysium, as described above, is actually composed of two separate membranes. The outermost membrane is referred to as the basement membrane, whereas the innermost layer is the plasma membrane or sarcolemma membrane. Know that the basement membrane is a loose collection of glycogen proteins with a collagen system and permeable to proteins, solutes, and other metabolites [6]. On the other hand, the plasma membrane functions as a true cell boundary, which may or may not be permeable to various substances. Despite this, from a regulatory standpoint, the plasma membrane utilizes a variety of transport mechanisms across the cell membrane [8].

Furthermore, the plasma membrane has unique features that are critical to the function of

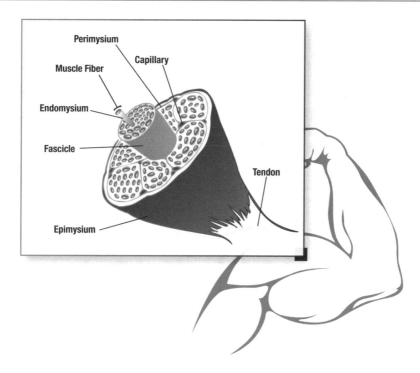

Fig. 3.2 Graphical representation of the three fascia layers. (Courtesy of Elizabeth A. Drum)

a muscle fiber. There are a series of shallow folds or indentations termed caveolae. These folds appear when the fiber is contracted or in a resting state, but disappear as the fiber is lengthened. During normal physical activity, the caveolae allow the muscle fibers to extend approximately 10–15 % without causing any damage to the fiber [9]. The plasma membrane also has a series of functional folds in the neuromuscular junction which help assist in the transmission of an action potential from the motor neuron to the muscle fiber. Finally, the plasma membrane is much more selective (vs. the basement membrane) to ions, solutes, and substrates crossing over, which contributes to the maintenance of acid–base balance [9]. The importance of acid–base balance relates to the proper functioning of skeletal muscle and its ability to continually produce force. For instance, if the internal muscle environment becomes too acidic, actin and myosin become "uncoupled" and force production is severely reduced, such as during a hard 5 km running race.

Satellite Cells

Another fascinating organizational element of skeletal muscle is the pervasive presence of satellite cells, known as myogenic stem cells, located between the basement and the plasma membranes of muscle fibers. These small cells were discovered by Alexander Mauro and named based on their peripheral location relative to the muscle fiber [10]. Primarily, satellite cells help initiate growth and development of existing and new muscle tissue along with promoting adaptations to training, injury, and disuse stimuli. Satellite cells have chemotaxis properties that are stimulated by muscle injury. When stimulated, satellite cells activate and proliferate, migrating to the damaged region. Satellite cells can move from their peripheral location outside the cell across the plasma membrane through the cytosol to the damaged region and fuse with existing myofibers (deep in the muscle cell) or differentiate to produce entirely new muscle cells [11]. The remarkable potential that satellite cells have

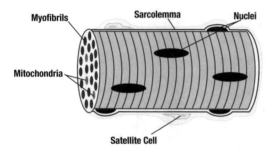

Fig. 3.3 Skeletal muscle *satellite cells* in relation to a single skeletal muscle fiber. (Courtesy of Elizabeth A. Drum)

in the recovery of muscle from injury is further explored in the following chapters. Figure 3.3 illustrates peripheral satellite cells in relation to a single muscle fiber.

Acknowledgments The authors warmly thank Elizabeth A. Drum for her time, efforts, and expertly drawn figures.

References

1. Lieber RL, Ward SR. Skeletal muscle design to meet functional demands. Phil Trans R Soc B. 2011;366:1466–76.
2. Ward SR, Eng CM, Smallwood LH, Lieber RL. Are current measurements of lower extremity muscle architecture accurate? Clin Orthop Relat Res. 2009;467:1074–82.
3. Lieber RL. Skeletal muscle structure, function and plasticity: the physiological basis of rehabilitation. 3rd ed. Baltimore: Lippincott Williams and Wilkins; 2010.
4. Kendall FP. Muscles: testing and function with posture and pain. 5th ed. Baltimore: Lippincott Williams & Wilkins; 2005.
5. Godon BCJ. Compartment syndrome and sport traumatology. Revue Medicale De Liege. 2005;60:109–16.
6. Sanes JR. The basement membrane/basal lamina of skeletal muscle. J Biol Chem. 2003;278:12601–4.
7. MacIntosh BR, Gardiner PF, McComas AJ. Skeletal muscle: form and function. Champaign: Human Kinetics; 2006.
8. McArdle WD, Katch FI, Katch VL. Exercise physiology: nutrition, energy, and human performance. 7th ed. Philadelphia: Wolters Kluwer/Lippincott Williams & Wilkins Health; 2010.
9. Brooks GA, Fahey TD, Baldwin KM. Exercise physiology: human bioenergetics and its applications. 4th ed. Boston: McGraw-Hill; 2005.
10. Mauro A. Satellite cell of skeletal muscle fibers. J Biophys Biochem Cytol. 1961;9:493–5.
11. Hawke TJ, Garry DJ. Myogenic satellite cells: physiology to molecular biology. J Appl Physiol. 2001;91:534–51.

Pathophysiology of Skeletal Muscle Injury

4

Andrew Swentik

Introduction

Muscle injuries are common problems that result in significant impairment of acute and chronic functions. An injury, for the purposes of this chapter, will be defined as a traumatic event that leads directly or indirectly to pain or loss of function. This definition provides a broad context in which the underlying principles, biomechanics, and pathophysiology of skeletal muscle injuries are reviewed in this chapter.

Skeletal muscle injuries occur owing to a variety of mechanisms. Fundamentally, a muscle injury occurs when the force applied to a muscle results in structural damage of the muscle tissue. The location, severity, and type of injury are dependent on the mechanism by which the force is applied, the condition of the tissue prior to injury, and the state of activation of the muscle during injury. Each of these factors plays an important role in determining the totality of any injury. Familiarity with the underlying mechanisms and variation in skeletal muscle injury is critical to the prevention, diagnosis, and treatment of these injuries. The objective of this chapter is to provide a scientific background and schema for understanding skeletal muscle injury as a basis for informing the specific discussion of muscle injuries in the posterior leg contained in the following chapters.

Principles of Skeletal Muscle Injury

Risk Factors

The complex nature of the musculoskeletal system, and the multiple interconnected movements needed to produce locomotion, lead to many possible areas of dysfunction that can increase the risk of muscle injury. When thinking broadly, any condition that limits the musculoskeletal system's ability to generate force or absorb energy has the potential to increase a person's risk of injury. This suggests a wide range of possible factors that may lead to an increased risk of injury (Textbox 4.1).

Textbox 4.1. Risk Factors for Muscle Injury

Factors related to an athlete's risk of muscle injury	
Fatigue	Conditioning
Weakness	Illness
Age	Gender
Medications/drugs	Nutritional status
Factors related to risk of injury to a specific muscle	
Muscles that cross two joints	
Muscles which function primarily in an eccentric manner	
Previously injured muscles	
Passively stretched muscles	

A. Swentik (✉)
Orthopedic Surgery, University of South Carolina, Columbia, SC, USA
e-mail: swentika@gmail.com

Underlying factors such as fatigue, weakness, and previous injury are often associated with muscle injury. Other commonly implicated risk factors include: poor conditioning, impaired nutritional status, age, gender, illness, mediations or illicit drugs, and skill level [1]. While these factors contribute to injury risk, their influence and contributions vary.

Eccentric contraction is also often noted as a cause for muscle injury, and it has been suggested muscles that function primarily in an eccentric manner are at greater risk for injury [1, 2]. A second group of muscles noted to be at an increased risk of injury are those which function across two joints. These two joint or biarthrodial muscles are through to be at increased risk of injury due to the fact that motion at one joint may place the muscle in a compromised position across the second, leading to an increased risk of injury [3]. Other muscles at risk for injury include previously injured muscles or those noted to have an imbalance between agonists and antagonists [3].

It is difficult to quantify the effect each factor has on overall risk, but due to the sheer volume of risk factors, it is easy to see why it is so difficult to develop comprehensive prevention programs and screening tests to eliminate the risk of muscle injuries in athletes and active people.

Types of Injuries

Injuries are typically classified with respect to the type, locations, and the severity of tissue damage. There is a variety of mechanisms that can produce injuries, and each produces a characteristic pathology. This specificity is the foundation for classifying muscle injuries by type. Muscle injuries can be further classified as either primary or secondary in nature. Primary injuries are a direct result of trauma to the muscle [3]. Examples of primary muscle injuries include lacerations, contusions, or strains. In contrast, secondary injuries have a delayed presentation, which results as a consequence of events set into place following the primary injury [4]. Secondary muscle injuries can follow directly from the evolution of the primary injury or be precipitated by compensations

made following the primary injury [1]. In addition, muscle injuries are also typically described as either acute or chronic in nature. The chronicity of any injury is an important determinant in the treatment and prognosis of a muscle injury.

Primary Injuries

Primary injuries are the most commonly seen type of injury. The pathophysiology of each primary injury is unique in its mechanism and its resulting pathology. Our discussion will focus on the three most common primary injuries in sports medicine: contusions, lacerations, and sprains (Textbox 4.2).

Textbox 4.2. Types of Muscle Injuries

Primary injuries
Strains
Contusions
Lacerations
Secondary injuries
Compartment syndromes
Delayed onset muscle soreness (DOMS)
Myositis ossificans

Contusion injuries are the result of blunt force trauma directed into the muscle. Contusions are typically characterized by hematoma formation and only minor superficial disruption of tissue [4]. The deeper, unnoticeable damage created in contusion injuries is often of greater concern than that notable on the surface. In lacerations, the insult is a more localized, sharp dissection of tissue. The damage incurred by tissue in lacerations is often more noticeable and visually impressive than those seen in blunt injuries. However, the true extent of injury in lacerations is often more localized and, therefore, may result in less structural damage than those seen in blunt injuries. However, in the setting of large or deep penetrating lacerations, the structural damage can be quite severe. The most commonly seen primary muscle injuries are muscle strains, which represent almost half of all athletic injuries [4]. Contributing factors to strains are the magnitude of force applied, rate of force application, and the mechanical strength of the muscle unit being tested [1]. Strains are classified based on the severity of tissue disruption, degree of dysfunction, and expected return to competition. Mild strains are those with minimal or no evidence of structural damage to the muscle. Strains that result in partial tearing of the muscle, but less than full thickness, are termed moderate. Severe strains are those with full or nearly full disruption of the muscle and are associated with marked impairment of function [1]. This muscle strain classification system is an attempt to simplify the continuum of strain injuries to aid in treatment decisions and help predict timing of expected recovery. Unfortunately, there remains significant variation within each group, and this limits the clinical utility of the classification system in attempts to make more nuanced assessments.

Secondary Injuries

The delayed presentation of secondary injuries can make their diagnosis more challenging than primary injuries. Examples of secondary injuries include compartment syndromes, delayed onset muscle soreness (DOMS), and myositis ossificans. This group also includes injuries that result secondary to alterations in a person's gait or movement patterns necessitated by compensations from the primary injury. The underlying theme in secondary injuries is that each injury is a consequence of some inciting event or pathology. Therefore, addressing secondary injuries requires identifying and optimizing treatment of the primary insult as well as addressing the secondary injury.

Compartment syndromes are characterized by pathologically increased tissue pressure within a confined space [4]. Compartment syndromes can be acute or chronic. One of the more common inciting events of acute compartment syndrome is severe blunt trauma. Blunt trauma has the potential to lead to compartment syndrome via fluid accumulation secondary to two different mechanisms. First, it may cause induction of the local inflammatory response following the traumatic event, leading to soft tissue swelling and edema. Secondly, if the trauma is severe enough, it may also cause direct compromise of vasculature

within the muscle, leading to bleeding and increased severity of the resulting edema [2]. Both mechanisms result in an increase in pressure within a confined space, leading to compression of the arterioles and an ischemic insult [4]. Acute compartment syndromes are considered an acute surgical emergency.

DOMS is a secondary injury seen following repeated eccentric contractions and is distinguished by its delayed onset. DOMS is typically noticed 12–24 h postexercise and typically peaks in intensity at 48 h [3–5]. It is described as a dull ache that increases in intensity with compression, stretching of the muscle, or contraction [6]. As the name suggests, it presents as soreness of the affected muscle and is often associated with reduced range of motion and stiffness. DOMS is classically seen following repetitive eccentric exercise or activity. DOMS usually is preceded by a notable loss of force development or exhaustion in the involved muscles exhibited during exercise. However, recent investigations have produced evidence to indicate the pathology responsible for the noted force deficit seen during eccentric exercise bouts is independent of the pathologic process responsible for DOMS [3]. The pathophysiology of DOMS is not well understood, with multiple theories currently being investigated. The cause of DOMS may be a combination of several proposed mechanisms. However, the sensitization of high-threshold mechanosensitve (HTM) receptors, the primary receptors for pressure-mediated pain in skeletal muscle, likely plays a major role. HTM receptors within skeletal muscle are typically in contact with the vascular bundles and have associations with the connective tissue but do not have direct contact with myofibers [5, 6]. The sensitivity of these receptors is increased by bradykinin and serotonin, both of which are commonly released from cells during an acute inflammatory reaction. The process responsible for the propagation and release of these sensitizing agents remains controversial. It is likely that the eccentric movements, which typically precede DOMS, create enough force on the muscle to cause a disruption within the muscle itself. The location of this disruption has at least two possible locations. Connective tissue and passive elements within the muscle play a critical role in the absorption of energy created during eccentric exercise and may become damaged following unaccustomed patterns of activity. Injury to these structures may induce local inflammatory responses responsible for initiating DOMS without disruption of the other muscle tissue elements [6]. Connective tissue damage as a cause, rather than damage to myofibers, is supported by the fact that markers of myofiber injury have not correlated well with the magnitude of DOMS in multiple studies. It has also been shown that there is a significant increase in urinary hydroxyproline, a breakdown product of collagen, in subjects suffering from DOMS [7]. However, direct myofiber injury has implicated as well and is supported by studies which have shown disruption and disorganization of myofibers of muscle in subjects with DOMS [6]. While the exact mechanism of DOMS remains elusive, continued investigations into the underlying pathology will have important clinical implications for athletes and active people.

As noted above, early force deficits noted following eccentric contractions were once thought to be induced by the same pathologic process as DOMS. However, studies have repeatedly demonstrated that as repetitions increased, the magnitude of the force deficit decreased, while the magnitude of DOMS and cellular pathology continue to increase [6]. Further support for differing mechanisms between observed alterations in task performance and the pathology causing DOMS is demonstrated through the finding that by increasing the interval time between repetitions, it is possible to prevent the histological changes typically seen with repeated eccentric contractions, without the ability to prevent significant loss of force generation [8]. Both of these findings indicate that the loss of function is likely the result of a local, transient, and reversible alteration within the cell. Probable explanations include disruption in the excitation–contraction coupling mechanism or the sarcomeres themselves, which lead to ineffective contractions [6].

Myositis ossificans is a condition seen following contusion injuries in which there is subsequent calcification of the muscle [4]. The arm and anterior thigh are the most common locations, a finding mostly likely due to the fact that those locations are the most common locations for severe contusion injuries [9]. One major risk factor for myositis ossificans is early reinjury to the muscle; this finding supports a theory of altered healing response as a possible mechanism for developing myositis ossificans. Unfortunately, the pathologic process underlying myositis ossificans is still not well understood, and it remains a secondary complication of muscle injury, resulting in significant morbidity with poor treatment options [4].

Chronic Injury

Although the focus of this chapter is primarily on acute injury, chronic injuries are an important classification of muscle injuries that have a differing pathophysiologic basis and resulting pathology. Chronic inflammation is often a result of repeated trauma or incomplete recovery from injury [1]. Tissues not fully recovered from an injury have the potential to enter a cycle of chronic inflammation and recurrent damage, secondary to the inflammation and/or degeneration. The hallmarks of chronic inflammation are mononuclear cells, tissue destruction, and fibrosis [10]. The proper treatment of acute injuries and full recovery prior to return of participation is one of the best ways to prevent chronic injuries. This highlights the critical role of acute injury management as the cornerstone of diagnosis, treatment, and prevention of muscle injuries more generally.

Injury Locations

Skeletal muscle injuries can be hard to predict and prevent. However, an understanding of skeletal muscle injury mechanisms and patterns can aid in diagnosis and prevention. The location and mechanism of laceration injuries is highly variable. However, skeletal muscle lacerations are most often caused by blunt traumas, such as a blow, collision, or fall, that penetrate deep tissue and muscle. Lower extremity lacerations account for about 13% of lacerations evaluated in the emergency department [11]. The overlying soft tissue of the posterior leg provides minimal protection for the underlying structures; so, it is important to consider injury to vessels, tendon, or nerve when evaluating laceration injuries in the posterior leg. Lacerations of the muscle may require surgical debridement, repair, and evacuation of hematoma or lavage. Several important structures in the posterior leg are at risk for laceration injury, most notably the Achilles tendon.

As mentioned, most of the lacerations seen involving the posterior leg are secondary to blunt trauma. This increases the risk of infection in these wounds for several reasons: first, because most of the traumatic lacerations result in irregularly shaped wounds, which have a high rate of contamination. The wounds are also at a higher risk of infection because the lower extremity has a decreased ability to heal wounds secondary to the increased hydrostatic pressure and resulting edema seen in traumatic wounds of this area [12]. It is important to note the immunization status of a patient with leg lacerations as the resulting contamination of the wound can introduce bacteria into the tissue, leading to a potential for tetanus. Due to the biomechanical importance of the posterior leg, as well as the increased risk of poor healing and infection, proper evaluation and treatment of leg lacerations is essential to avoid potential complications.

Muscle contusions are the second most common sports injury [13]. The severity and resulting limitations produced by contusions are more predictable and are direct products of the object and force which resulted in the trauma. These factors determine the degree of myofibril and vascular disruption and the size of the associated intramuscular hematoma. Contusion injuries initiate an immediate cascade of pathophysiologic changes, and the initial management approach focuses on limiting hematoma formation, further muscle damage, and potential complications such as compartment syndrome or myositis ossificans.

While lacerations and contusion injuries are unpredictable and located at the site of trauma, strain injuries typically occur at consistent locations within the muscle. The myotendinous junction (MTJ) has been well established as the principal site of acute muscle strains [1–4, 6]. The severity of strain injuries is dependent on the magnitude of force applied, rate of force application, and strength of the musculotendinous structures involved [6]. Studies of strain injuries have also highlighted the difference between passively stretched and activated muscle. These studies consistently demonstrate that there is no difference in the muscle length at failure between passive and stimulated muscles [6]. However, the amount of force required prior to failure has been shown to be 15–30% higher, and the amount of energy that a muscle is able to absorb is estimated to be around 100% higher in stimulated muscles when compared to muscles passively stretched to failure [1, 14, 15]. In both stimulated and passive muscles, the site of failure is consistently the MTJ, although there are subtle differences in the exact location of failure depending on the activation status of the muscle. Using electron microscopy, Tidball was able to show actively stimulated muscles fail at the proximal MTJ just external to the membrane, with no soft tissue still attached. This is in contrast to the disruption occurring at the z-disk just distal to the proximal MTJ seen in passive muscle failure [14]. So, while the general location of strain injuries is consistent at the MTJ, there is some predictable variability in the structural components which failed, depending on the state of muscle activation at the time of injury.

Biomechanics of Injury

Biomechanical properties of the musculoskeletal system are functionally important in injuries. An understanding of the force distribution in motion and the ability of muscles to generate force is essential when attempting to determine the nature of muscle injuries. Beginning with the functional units of muscle, their organization, and supporting tissue will allow us to proceed into force production and energy absorption, and help us understand the fundamental properties of injury.

Organization

The function of the musculoskeletal system is dependent on its structural organization. The structure, organization, and physiology of the musculoskeletal system were the focus of the preceding chapters, but here we will review a few important properties critical to the pathophysiology of muscle injuries (Textbox 4.3).

Textbox 4.3. General Outline of Muscle Structure

Contractile unit: Sarcomere	
Functional unit: Muscle fiber	Composed of sarcomeres arranged in series
Muscle fiber arrangement	Parallel: Fusiform, Fan, Strap
	Pennate: Unipennate, Bipennate, Multipennate

We will begin by reviewing the functional unit of muscle: the muscle fiber. The important detail of a muscle fiber is the simple fact that it is composed of multiple sarcomeres, which are the smallest contractile unit of muscle [1, 4]. Individual muscle fibers are bundled together into fascicles and arranged in various patterns. The different arrangements include parallel or pennate structures, which each have significantly different biomechanical properties. Parallel muscles can be subclassified as fusiform, fan, or strap muscles, while pennate muscles can be unipennate, bipennate, or multipennate in form. Muscles are innervated by α motor neurons that are organized into motor units controlling specific muscle fibers throughout the muscle. A motor unit consists of anywhere between 10 and more than 1000 muscle fibers, distributed throughout the muscle [4]. It is believed that the neuron itself plays an important role in determining fiber type, with each neuron innervating a homogenous population of fibers. The arrangement of sarcomeres, pattern of muscle fiber alignment, and individual motor units all impart specific biomechanical properties into muscles and are important determinants in the functional capabilities of a given muscle and also the risk for injury in that muscle.

Force Production

Force generation is a complicated process, which is dependent not only on the biomechanical properties of muscle but the manner in which they are activated. The central nervous system is able to vary the input into muscles using temporal or spatial summation. Temporal summation alters force production by increasing the frequency of neuron firing, while spatial summation is accomplished by increasing the number of motor units recruited. Spatial summation's use is limited to forces less than 50 % of maximum force generation, after which temporal summation is required [4]. The modulation of muscle activation by these summation strategies allows for the efficient generation of force to effectively carry out our daily activities.

Also important to the discussion of muscle injuries are the biomechanical properties of muscle that influence force production. The length–tension and force–velocity properties of muscle help illustrate the importance of muscle structure. The amount of force a muscle is capable of producing is proportional to the number of cross-bridges in parallel. The length–tension principle states that as the length of a muscle is altered from its optimal cross-bridge length, the muscle will have a resulting decrease in ability to produce force [1]. This relationship is ultimately the result of a decrease in the number of cross-bridges available as the muscle changes length [1]. The force–velocity relationship states that as the velocity of muscle contractions increases, its ability to generate force decreases [1]. As mentioned, the sarcomeres in a muscle fiber are arranged in series, while the unique pennate arrangement of muscles is akin to adding muscle fibers in parallel within the muscle. Adding cross-bridges in series is important for increasing velocity production, while adding them in parallel will increase force generation. We now have a basic understanding of a muscle's ability to generate force, and a moderate assessment of its risk for injury, by noting the location of muscle, the number of joints crossed, and the fiber arrangement.

Energy Absorption

Force production is important, but a muscle's ability to absorb energy also plays an important role in injuries. Muscle has both active and passive properties, which are involved in energy absorption. Passive properties are determined by the connective tissue contained within the muscle and are independent of the state of activation of the muscle. The passive component of energy absorption is a function of all noncontractile proteins found within the muscle, including collagen, sarcomeres, and even the endomysium [3]. Passive properties of the muscle are also important in distribution of tension within a muscle [1]. Active properties of muscle are determined by the contractile units, and their ability to absorb energy is highly dependent on the state of activation. Active muscle will absorb 100 % more energy prior to failure than passively stretched muscle [3, 14]. This increase in ability to absorb energy plays an important role in our ability to protect ourselves from injury. This structural property of muscle explains the common observation that injuries often occur when the individual is caught off guard by a sudden application of force or change in body position.

Pathophysiology of Skeletal Muscle Injury

Anyone who has ever experienced or carefully observed a muscle injury can attest to hallmarks of inflammation as famously described by Roman physician and polymath Aulus Cornelius Celsus, "rubor et tumor cum calore et dolore." Or redness and swelling with heat and pain. Al-though our fundamental intuitions and observations of the pathophysiology of muscle injury are long standing, our knowledge of the details underlying these intuitions and observations continues to expand. Scientific investigation has led to a detailed account of the local and global changes that occur post injury. Although there are commonalities in the major cellular players, the timing of events, and even some of the chemical mediators responsible in injuries generally, it is now clear that each tissue and each type of injury has its own unique pathophysiology. While our knowledge of these differences is important, it remains helpful to understand the pathophysiology of injury generally in the broad categories of inflammation, repair, and remodeling.

Inflammatory Phase

The inflammatory response begins immediately after injury. The induction of the inflammatory response will vary depending on the mechanism of injury. Inflammation is generally considered as resulting from the coordinated response between blood vessels, local tissues, and leukocytes, consisting of a change in blood vessel diameter, structural changes in the vasculature, and leukocyte recruitment to the site of injury [10]. Vasoactive mediators including nitrous oxide (NO), bradykinin, serotonin, and histamine help to produce the predictable signs and symptoms of early inflammation [3] (Table 4.1).

The tearing of the local tissue and blood vessels incites the inflammatory response by releasing localized extracellular matrix (ECM)-bound growth factors [2]. Inflammatory cytokines from the vascular system are also released into the

Table 4.1 Initiation of the inflammatory phase

Local tissue response	Primary cells	Signaling molecules	Timing
Local edema	PMNs	NO	From time of injury to 48–72 h[a]
Local injury induces vasodilation	Macrophages	Bradykinin	
Increased vascular permeability	Mast cells	Serotonin	
Leukocyte activation and attraction	Platelets	Histamine	

PMNs polymorphonuclear leukocyte, *NO* nitrous oxide

[a] Exact timing of inflammatory phase is highly variable and dependent on the type of injury as well as the subsequent treatment

injured area. A vascular response quickly follows and includes a transient vasoconstriction and subsequent vasodilatation. The primary mediators of the vasodilation are histamine and NO. The vasodilation is accompanied by an increase in vascular permeability mediated by bradykinin, substance P, histamine, and leukotrienes [10]. The change in vascular membrane permeability allows rapid migration of leukocytes, as well as other inflammatory mediators, and is one of the major causes of edema that follows muscle injuries.

Edema caused by changes in vascular permeability is often accompanied by significant vascular disruption and development of an acute hematoma. Expansion of the hematoma is limited by fibrin clot formation and local tissue characteristics that lead to tamponade. Structural damage caused by the injury is also limited by development of a contraction band or membrane that occurs as part of the local tissue necrosis. This process was best demonstrated by Hurme et al. who noted, "The advancing necrotic front was demarcated by the formation of a new membrane" [16]. Formation of this membrane, subsequently coined a contraction band, early in the injury process is an important barrier in controlling the damage produced by injury. By containing the hematoma through these mechanisms, a microenvironment is created that allows the healing process to progress and be coordinated at a local level.

Following the acute phase response is the recruitment and activation of leukocytes. This stage is propagated by multiple different cells and stored cytokines typically held in an inactive state within the ECM [2]. Other chemical mediators are locally produced or released from circulating neutrophils, macrophages, mast cells, or even platelets [10]. Typically, bone marrow cells such as polymorphonuclear leukocytes (PMNs) have begun to divide and are found as quickly as 1 h post-injury. PMNs are the predominate cells found at the site of injury for the first 24–48 h, at which time macrophages begin to outnumber neutrophils [2, 10, 17, 18]. Studies have demonstrated that there are at least two specific populations of macrophages seen in healing of muscle

injuries. The first become evident in wounds within 24 h of injury. They play an important role not only in organization of the wound but in activation and promotion of myogenic cells. These macrophages are noted by the expression of cluster of differentiation 68 (CD68) and the noted absence of CD163. They are believed to play a large role in phagocytosis and induction of pro-inflammatory cytokines such as tumor necrosis factor (TNF)-α and interleukin (IL)-1β. They are replaced by the second phase of macrophage invasion, cells noted to be CD68-negative and CD163-positive, beginning 48 h or more post injury. Their function is different from that of the early macrophages as they typically secrete cytokines such as IL-10 and function in more of an anti-inflammatory than pro-inflammatory role [19]. This second wave of macrophages is also believed to release cytokines that enhance myogenic proliferation and differentiation. The transition from PMNs to macrophages is aided by the fact that PMNs have shorter life than macrophages, and unlike macrophages, they don't seem to replicate in tissues during this process [10], making the transition a necessary and functionally important element in the healing process.

The coordination and activation of leukocytes is a complex process that has become a focus area for potential treatment interventions. As leukocytes are attracted to the area of inflammation, cytokines produced by tissue macrophages, endothelial cells, or mast cells help attach leukocytes to damaged endothelial cells. The first major family of proteins involved in leukocyte adhesion is selectins. Selectins are weak binders of leukocytes but are very effective in slowing the leukocytes down enough to allow integrins to bind more firmly and trap leukocytes locally. TNF-α and IL-1β are two primary cytokines produced to increase integrin expression and are, thus, the primary cytokines involved in leukocyte recruitment [10]. The relationship between TNF-α and integrins will also be very important in the healing process seen later as integrins are a group of proteins involved in multiple biological processes [2]. Alterations of both TNF-α and IL-1β are being investigated as targets for therapeutic intervention.

Once localized to the site of injury, leukocytes must then cross the endothelial membrane. As mentioned earlier, multiple substances are produced locally to alter the permeability of the membrane. In addition to those vasoactive mediators, chemokines are produced that create a chemical gradient down which leukocytes migrate, thereby ensuring concentrations of these cells in the area of injury. Chemoattractants produced in this process include IL-8, complement components, and leukotriene (LT)B4 [10].

The final step in leukocyte recruitment is activation. There are multiple ways leukocytes are activated. Specific receptors expressed, termed toll-like receptors (TLRs), bind to and activate leukocytes. In addition, nonviable tissue is marked for phagocytosis in a process called opsonization. Natural killer cells or T cells produce opsonins, which are attached to particles or cells in need of removal. The opsonins are then bound by specific receptors expressed on leukocytes, inducing phagocytosis. A third process of leukocyte activation involves receptors expressed on leukocytes, which are specific for other cytokines produced during the injury process. One such cytokine is interferon (INF)-γ. INF-γ is considered the major macrophage-activating cytokine produced [10]. These various methods are all thought to play a critical role in activating leukocytes to induce effective phagocytosis to remove cellular debris.

The process of phagocytosis by leukocytes is carried out by chemicals produced inside macrophages or neutrophils. Reactive oxygen species (ROS) and reactive nitrogen species are the most common compounds produced. Major enzymes that generate the active compounds include nicotinaminde adenine dinucleaotide phosphate (NADPH) oxidase and myloperoxidase (MPO). NADPH oxidase is responsible for reducing oxygen and creating superoxide anions. MPO is utilized in the production of hypochlorite when in the presence of Cl^- and H_2O_2. NO is commonly involved in these processes as well as in the creation of nitrogen-containing reactive species such as peroxynitrite (ONOO·) [10, 20]. The ROS and reactive nitrogen species produced are then utilized following phagocytosis of the damaged tissue. The removal of nonviable cells and cellular debris from the site of injury prepares the area, allowing the repair phase to proceed fully.

Repair Phase

The repair phase actually begins soon after the injury. Repair involves a balance between two opposing processes; the formation of a connective tissue scar and regeneration of myofibers. These processes coincide, collide, and yet, must work collaboratively to heal the injured muscle (Textbox 4.4).

Textbox 4.4. Repair Phase

Repair phase balances the production of granulation tissue and development of myogenic cells	
Granulation tissue	Fibrin and fibronectin help with early stabilization
	Type III collagen is initially produced and then slowly replaced by type I collagen
	Some motion across the developing scar is needed to increase tensile strength
	Granulation tissue is the weakest area of healing tissue for the first 10 days[a]
Muscle repair	Satellite cells are the primary cells responsible for myocyte replacement and repair. They are cells located between the sarcolemma and the basal lamina
	Other cells capable of myogenic potential are identifiable by the expression of Pax-7
	Satellite cell activation is via delta-1 ligand activation of the Notch signaling pathway
	Notch activation then stimulates the production of the myogenic regulatory factors (MRFs)
	MyoD and Mfy5—regulate satellite cell proliferation and specification into myocytes
	MyoG and MRF4—regulate cell differentiation and control the cell cycle
	Duration: muscle repair phase lasts 2–3 weeks

[a] Granulation tissue, or the healing tissue is still significantly weaker than the muscle fibers for the first ten days and repeat trauma will cause failure in this area.

Traditionally, treatment approaches have aimed at decreasing connective tissue scar formation in an attempt to increase myofiber formation and hasten the recovery process. However, recently, it has become clear that these two processes are intertwined and both are necessary for optimal healing. The interconnection between the two processes is still not completely understood; however, recent studies have begun to unravel some of the clinically relevant connections that exist.

Cytokines are produced from many of the same cells that help to induce the acute inflammatory response. Bloodborne inflammatory cells, such as macrophages and fibroblasts, are major producers of important cytokines such as transforming growth factor (TFG-β), IL-1β, IL-6, insulin-like growth factor (IGF), fibroblast growth factor (FGF), or TNF-α) [2]. These cytokines are also commonly seen within the ECM of healthy muscle. This helps explain why one of the determining factors in the healing process is the state of the basement membrane as disruption of the basement membrane allows the release of those tissue-specific growth factors. The result is a locally produced, highly coordinated response that is specific to each tissue and each type of injury.

While the inflammatory response is working to clear disrupted tissue from wounds, the repair process has begun. Before myocytes begin the repair of damaged myofibers, fibroblasts have begun to stabilize the wound. As mentioned, the wound debridement performed is highly specific, sparing the basal lamia so it can act as an early scaffold for wound stabilization. Fibrin and fibronectin produce granulation tissue to fill in the defect [2, 10]. As fibroblasts arrive, they produce proteins and proteoglycans found in the native ECM. Through the fibroblast production of ECM proteins, the local environment of the wound is altered to resemble the pre-injury state. Because one of the major inducers of the inflammatory cascade is disruption of the basement membrane, early stabilization of this environment may play an important role in limiting the inflammatory response and the transition to the repair phase. Two important proteins synthesized by fibroblasts are

fibronectin and tenascin-C. These two proteins form multimeric fibers that add strength and elastic properties to the wound. Type III collagen is the primary form of collagen produced after injury. Type III collagen creates a large bulky scar but one that is generally successful in stabilizing the wound. Over the next few days, type I collagen is produced, and the scar contracts in size. The tensile strength of the wound increases during this period, secondary to cross-linking of collagen. This process takes time, and the scar is at its weakest point for approximately the first 10 days post injury [2, 10, 19].

Following stabilization of the wound by fibroblasts and scar formation, the wound undergoes a process to repair the injured muscle. This requires, first and foremost, the activation of satellite cells. Satellite cells are a quiescent population of cells located between the sarcolemma and the basal lamina, and are the primary cells responsible for myocyte replacement and repair [19]. Cells capable of myogenic potential are identifiable by the expression of specific cellular markers. The most common is Pax-7, seen in almost all cells with myogenic potential; others include CD 34 and M-cadherin [19]. The process of satellite cell activation is an active area of research and has significant clinical implications because of the inherent potential to develop novel treatments for muscle injury.

Two of the pathways shown to be influential in satellite cell activation are the Wnt and Notch signaling pathways. Their activation is accomplished via Delta-1 ligand activation of the Notch signaling pathway, resulting in an activation of a family of muscle-specific transcription factors or MRFs [19]. Once activated, the MRFs control proliferation, specification, and differentiation of satellite cells. Another key growth factor currently being investigated is IGF. The pathways and specific role of IGF in satellite cell activation are still not completely understood, but it has been demonstrated that there are several different IGFs which seem to be involved in the process. IGF-I has been shown to influence both proliferation and differentiation, while IGF-II's effects seem more localized to the differentiation phase [19].

The proliferation of myogenic cells begins when the *Pax-7* gene is activated. Once activated, MRFs control the progression of satellite cells through the cell cycle. Two MRFs, MyoD and Myf5, are influential early in the cell cycle and appear to be particularly important in regulation of proliferation and specification. Myogenin or MyoG and Mrf4 are seen in the later phases of the cell cycle, and their primary influence is on differentiation and termination of the cell cycle [19, 21]. Each transcription factor is expressed in a timing-dependent fashion to guide the replication process. Following the activation of Pax-7, a rapid downstream increase in the translation of *Myf-5* genes is seen, initiating the cell cycle. As the cycle progresses, the next MRF expressed is Myo-D. Myo-D is believed to be the key myogenic transcription factor, controlling the cells' ability to transcribe cell cycle transcription factors. Myogenic proteins share a highly conserved basic helix–loop–helix (bHLH) binding domain, and activation requires binding to the muscle-specific E-box consensus sequence [19]. It has been shown that one of the key regulatory mechanisms is access to this E-box sequence. Myo-D's ability to open the chromatin structure is essential in allowing other transcription factors access to areas on the chromatin structure that are otherwise not available [21]. As with most regulatory factors, the exact signaling mechanisms and downstream effects of Myo-D appear to fluctuate depending on environment and phase of the cell cycle. Despite that, its expression is believed to be responsible for specification of satellite cells into myoblasts. Myo-D is also a key factor in the expression of Myo-g, the transcription factor most responsible for differentiation of myoblasts. Activation of Myo-g is responsible for exit from the cell cycle and the formation of myotubules. The open chromatin structure established early in the cell cycle is a key determinant in the ability of Myo-g to function as it is a strong activator of transcription in this state. The combined activity of Myo-D and Myo-g helps to induce the expression of MRF-4, directing maturation of myotubules and formation myofilaments [21]. The end result of this process is multinucleated fibers that become mature muscle fibers.

The stimulation of satellite cells and each pathway described to this point have multiple factors influencing their progression. Our understanding of the signaling mechanisms and molecules responsible for regulation, progression, and intercommunication between these pathways is an area of active research. Several other growth factors believed to be influential in the process include platelet-derived growth factor (PDGF), FGF, and hepatocyte growth factor (HGF).

Once satellite cells have formed regenerating myofibers, they begin to branch off from injury sites. Early in the repair process the cells remain unattached and progressively grow toward the newly formed scar. During this process, they add stability to the wound with secondary attachments they make to the ECM on their lateral border [2]. Once the ends of the myofibers have successfully reached the scar, attachments are created in a similar manner as typically seen at myotendinous junctions. Once attachments are made to the scar, the muscle functions as two separate units connected in series [2]. Over time, the scar thickness decreases and the two muscle fibers are brought closer together. There are several requirements for this process to happen successfully. The first is stress on the wound. For lateral attachments between myofibers and the ECM, some stress across the wound is needed, helping to explain why it may be important to limit excessive immobilization following injuries [2, 3]. For full recovery, the muscle must also reestablish innervation and revascularization of the muscle on each side of the scar. Early in the process, newly formed myotubes are deficient in mitochondria and rely heavily on anaerobic metabolism for growth. However, aerobic metabolism becomes a requirement as healing progresses and the myofibers begin to function as mature multinucleated cells [3].

The repair phase typically lasts 2–3 weeks. During this time, the injured area and the newly formed scar are the weakest point for the first 10 days following the injury. However, after 10 days, the scar has stabilized the wound sufficiently that if reinjury occurs, it is typically noted to be found within muscle tissue surrounding the original injury. Understanding of this process provides some basis to inform clinical recommendations regarding post-injury activity to maximize the healing process [2].

Remodeling Phase

The repair and remodeling phases overlap as the muscle continues to heal. The exact transition is difficult to pinpoint and probably is different depending on the perspective of the examiner. Clinically, the repair phase is typically considered to be complete once there is no noticeable inflammation and pain-free range of motion is obtained [3]. While in the laboratory research setting, the transition to the remodeling phase is based on the observation of further ECM deposition and initiation of tissue remodeling [10]. Regardless of the point of transition, full remodeling of injuries is a slow process that begins while the repair phase is active and can take weeks to months or even longer depending on the severity of the injury. Each tissue component within the muscle must undergo remodeling before the healing process is considered complete. For example, the connective tissue scar will continue to evolve, secondary to changing collagen structures. The amount of type III collagen continues to decrease and be replaced by type I fibers. Throughout the remodeling phase, the type I collagen also continues to strengthen via formation of cross-links and increased fiber size. A set of enzymes influential in the remodeling of connective tissue are matrix metalloproteinases (MMPs), found in the ECM. MMPs are a family of enzymes that include collagenases and stromelysins, and are involved in the degradation of collagen and fibronectin, allowing the scar size to be progressively decreased as the strength of the wound increases [10]. Remodeling and reorganization of the muscle itself also continues throughout the remodeling phase. The increased vascularity seen in the inflammatory and repair phases by this point has largely resolved, and the hyperemic appearance of the tissue resolves [3].

Clinical Application of Research

Reviewing the current clinical management for musculoskeletal injuries in light of the basic science research demonstrates how far our understanding of optimal treatment can still progress. A primary goal of any clinically relevant research program is to illuminate the underlying processes so that this understanding can be used to improve health and function. The research on muscle pathophysiology holds particular promise for clinical applications and improved outcomes. Current research has successfully demonstrated the importance of each phase of the healing process and demonstrated why treatments limiting any one phase produce suboptimal results. There is a need to translate the current knowledge of muscle injuries into the clinical care of patients and perform clinical studies to assess the effect these approaches have on outcomes. In addition, continued research efforts should provide promise for the development of new modalities that could revolutionize the care of muscle injuries.

Summary

Musculoskeletal injuries are complex. There are a variety of risk factors that influence the location, severity, and resulting limitations. The three most common primary injuries are contusions, lacerations, and strains. Of those three, acute strains account for over half of the injuries seen in athletes. Muscles that cross two joints or are active during eccentric movements are at greater risk for strain injury. Not only are primary injuries a concern but secondary injuries can be very impactful to athletes. Although the pathophysiology of the most common secondary injury, DOMS, is not well known, its self-limiting nature makes its long-term impact less severe. The structural makeup of the musculoskeletal system has a large influence in the biomechanics of our movement, which makes understanding it essential to the development and implementation of treatments.

Our knowledge of the pathophysiology of muscle injury is rapidly expanding. Muscle injury follows the well-described process seen in healing of many different types of tissue—inflammation, repair, and remodeling. The more we learn about the inflammation phase, the more it becomes clear that this phase sets the stage for repair and remodeling to follow. Satellite cells are the primary cells responsible for regeneration of myofibers and allow healing of injured muscle. MRFs are a group of transcription factors, which regulate the cell cycle of activated satellite cells, and are a major focus of current research. Remodeling of the injury plays an important role in returning to full function; however, many of the final limitations of the injury are already determined prior to the remodeling ever starting. Limiting the damage caused by inflammation and minimizing scar formation can be keys to improving healing, but they must be done without causing negative downstream effects mediated by signaling pathways that control repair and remodeling.

References

1. Whiting WC, Zernicke RF. Biomechanics of musculoskeletal injury. 2nd ed. Chelsea: Sheridan Books; 2008.
2. Järvinen TA, Järvinen TL, Kääriäinen M, Kalima H, Järvinen M. Muscle injuries biology and treatment. Am J Sports Med. 2005;33:745–64.
3. Page P. Pathophysiology of acute exercise-induced muscular injury: clinical implications. J Athl Train. 1995;30(1):29–34.
4. DeLee JC, Drez D Jr, Miller MD. DeLee & Drez's orthopaedic sports medicine principles and practice. 3rd ed. Philadelphia: Saunders; 2010.
5. Lewis PB, Ruby D, Bush-Joseph CA. Muscle soreness and delayed-onset muscle soreness. Clin Sports Med. 2012;31(2):255–62.
6. Magee DJ, Manske RC, Zachazewski JE, Quillen WS. Athletic and sport issues in musculoskeletal rehabilitation. St Louis: Elsevier; 2011.
7. Abraham WM. Factors in delayed muscle soreness. Med Sci Sports. 1977;9(1):11–20.
8. Stauber WT, Willems ME. Prevention of histopathologic changes from 30 repeated stretches of active rat skeletal muscles by long inter-stretch rest times. Eur J Appl Physiol. 2002;88(1–2):94–9.
9. Wiesel BB, Sankar WN, Delahay JN, Wiesel SW. Orthopaedic surgery principles of diagnosis and treatment. Philadelphia: Lippincott Williams and Wilkins; 2011.
10. Robbins SL, Kumar V, Cotran RS. Robbins and Cotran pathologic basis of disease. 8th ed. Philadelphia: Saunders; 2010.
11. Singer AJ, Thode HC Jr, Hollander JE. National trends in ED lacerations between 1992 and 2002. Am J Emerg Med. 2006;24(2):183–8.
12. Quinn JV, Polevoi SK, Kohn MA. Traumatic lacerations: what are the risks for infection and has the 'golden period' of laceration care disappeared? Emerg Med J. 2014;31(2):96–100.
13. Beiner JM, Jokl P. Muscle contusion injuries: current treatment options. J Am Acad Orthop Surg. 2001;9(4):227–37.
14. Tidball JG, Salem G, Zernicke R. Site and mechanical conditions for failure of skeletal muscle in experimental strain injuries. J Appl Physiol. 1993;74(3):1280–6.
15. Garrett WE Jr, Safran MR, Seaber AV, Glisson RR, Ribbeck BM. Biomechanical comparison of stimulated and nonstimulated skeletal muscle pulled to failure. Am J Sports Med. 1987;15(5):448–54.
16. Hurme T, Kalimo H, Lehto M, Järvinen M. Healing of skeletal muscle injury: an ultrastructural and immunohistochemical study. Med Sci Sports Exerc. 1991;23(7):801–10.
17. Pinniger GJ, Lavin T, Bakker A. Skeletal muscle weakness caused by carrageenan-induced inflamation. Muscle Nerve. 2012;46:413–20.
18. Supinski GS, Callahan LA. Free radical-mediated skeletal muscle dysfunction in inflammatory conditions. J Appl Physiol. 2007;102:2056–63.
19. Zanou N, Gailly P. Skeletal muscle hypertrophy and regeneration: interplay between the myogenic regulatory factors (MRFs) and insulin-like growth factors (IGFs) pathways. Cell Mol Life Sci. 2013;70:4117–30. Epub ahead of print accessed at pubmed.gov.
20. Ghaly A, Marsh D. Ischaemia-reperfusion modulates inflammation and fibrosis of skeletal muscle after contusion injury. Int J Exp Path. 2010;91:244–55.
21. Singh K, Dilworth JF. Differential modulation of cell cycle progression distinguishes members of the myogenic regulatory factor family of transcription factors. FEBS J. 2013;280:3991–4003. Epub ahead of print accessed at pubmed.gov.

Neurophysiology of Musculoskeletal Pain

5

Erich N. Ottem

Introduction

Musculoskeletal disorders are the leading causes of clinically relevant pain in every population globally. Thus, musculoskeletal pain is a major medical condition that negatively affects a significant percentage of the worldwide population. A recent study of patients with musculoskeletal disorders in the USA found they incur annual medical care costs of approximately US$240 billion, of which US$77 billion is directly related to musculoskeletal pain management [1]. A comprehensive series of studies found that at any given time, 20–30% of European adults are affected by musculoskeletal pain, and lower back pain, specifically, is experienced by 60–85% of individuals over their lifetime [2–4]. In another research report, 37% of males and 65% of females randomly selected from a population of 1504 adults aged 30–60 displayed signs and symptoms of musculoskeletal pain [5]. Despite its prevalence and the physical, psychological, and economic burden surrounding the disorder, research and medical communities are, to date, lacking a thorough understanding of many of the underlying mechanisms generating pain from musculoskeletal origins. Highlighting these deficits, the International Association for the Study of Pain

(IASP) recently identified three current clinical challenges associated with musculoskeletal pain:

- Treatment for musculoskeletal pain is not adequate.
- At the chronic level, musculoskeletal pain is typically managed, but not cured.
- It is often difficult to relate pathophysiological changes to the patient's actual pain, which makes musculoskeletal pain especially challenging to diagnose.

This chapter aims to summarize our current understanding of the physical manifestation of musculoskeletal pain, the cellular, molecular, and neurological origins of musculoskeletal pain conduction, and some current treatment strategies that may mitigate the widespread and debilitating disorder.

Musculoskeletal Pain: Common Clinical Presentations

In the last few decades, the research and medical communities' understanding of the nature and origin of pain has vastly improved. Clinicians and primary researchers now understand that the sensation of pain arises from several different tissue types and, as such, is triggered by numerous molecular mechanisms and neural pathways. Accordingly, the perception, or quality, of pain is interpreted in many different ways,

E. N. Ottem (✉)
Department of Biology, Northern Michigan University, Marquette, MI, USA
e-mail: eottem@nmu.edu

Table 5.1 Comparison of pain presentation: cutaneous and visceral pain versus musculoskeletal pain

	Perception of pain	Pain tolerance	Pain referral
Cutaneous and visceral pain	Sharp, pricking, burning, and/or cutting sensations	Easily or moderately tolerated	No pain referral and no secondary hyperalgesia
Musculoskeletal pain	Aching and cramping	Poorly tolerated	Often accompanied by pain referral and secondary hyperalgesia

depending on the point and mechanism of origin. Cutaneous and visceral pain, for example, is typified by sharp, pricking, burning, and/or cutting sensations. Additionally, cutaneous and visceral pain is easily localized and does not display a propensity for referral to other tissues or somatic locations. In general, cutaneous and visceral pain is moderately to easily tolerated [6]. In contrast, musculoskeletal pain is characterized by sensations of aching and cramping which are difficult to localize, poorly tolerated, and frequently exhibit referral to deep somatic tissues, such as other muscle groups, fascia, and joints [7–9]. Prolonged musculoskeletal pain associated with focal muscle damage or injury is also associated with an increased incidence of secondary hyperalgesia, or the spreading of chronic pain to undamaged, uninjured muscle. The basic differences between musculoskeletal pain and cutaneous and visceral pain are summarized in Table 5.1. Importantly, the degree of musculoskeletal pain intensity and its duration both influence the degree of muscular hyperalgesia over time [10–12]. Below, we discuss three common disorders involving musculoskeletal pain.

Musculoskeletal Pain Associated with Muscle Injury

Pain arising from damaged muscle is classified as either acute or chronic. Macro- or microtrauma, along with mechanical overload of muscles during contraction or stretch phases, is the most common cause of acute musculoskeletal pain [13]. Common muscle soreness, or type I muscle strain, arising from mechanical overload or overuse experienced following exercise or work-related actions is typically perceived during or immediately following activity. The duration of this type of musculoskeletal soreness is transient,

generally lasts for only hours, and is coupled with muscle stiffness and tenderness [13, 14]. Distinct from the symptoms associated with type I muscle strain, delayed onset muscle soreness (DOMS) describes musculoskeletal pain that develops up to 24 h *after* overactivity or muscular overload. As DOMS progresses, musculoskeletal pain, weakness, and stiffness steadily increase in intensity and peak within 2–3 days following onset. Due to underlying cellular damage and ongoing inflammatory processes (discussed later in this chapter) related to the acute muscle damage associated with DOMS, full recovery of muscle function may take weeks to occur [14].

The proximal causes underlying chronic musculoskeletal pain following overload or overuse are somewhat more difficult to identify. Often, it is the accumulation of muscle trauma or repeated acute muscle damage that leads to the onset of chronic musculoskeletal pain which is often accompanied by hyperalgesia [13]. There are several musculoskeletal and neuromuscular disorders (most outside the scope of this chapter) that include symptomatic chronic muscular pain. Two disorders with associated chronic musculoskeletal pain are described below.

Musculoskeletal Pain Associated with Myofascial Pain Syndrome

Both hyperalgesia and referred pain of muscular origin are hallmarks of a musculoskeletal pain condition known as myofascial pain syndrome (MPS) and highlight the unique nature of the myosensory pathway. MPS is caused by the appearance of myofascial trigger points (TrPs) located within muscles. Activated by chronic or acute muscular overload or overuse, TrPs are defined as "taut bands" of muscle fibers that extend the length of the entire muscle and are chronically contracted [15–18]. Interestingly, the constant contracted state of these taut bands is independent of typical presynaptic motor neuron activity and subsequent end-plate action potential generation. Instead, chronic contraction of the taut bands seems to originate via abnormal acetylcholine release and subsequent extremely high-frequency miniature end-plate potential activity [15–18]. Activated TrPs, which create multiple taut bands within a muscle or muscles, subsequently lead to the formation of areas known as zones of tenderness which are associated with regions of hypoxia. It is the creation of these zones of tenderness that gives rise to sensory musculoskeletal pain associated with MPS. The area of TrP formation becomes hypersensitive to stimulation and normally nonpainful stimuli become painful (allodynia). The immediate consequence of TrP formation in an affected muscle is increased fatigability, pain during contraction, and a restriction of range of motion. Additionally, the pain associated with TrP formation is referred to other muscle groups, distinct from the locally affected muscle [15–18]. Progressive musculoskeletal pain associated with spreading hyperalgesia is a common occurrence associated with MPS due, in part, to TrP formation in compensating muscles or abnormally contracted postural muscles [16]. Later in this chapter, we will discuss potential mechanisms which may underlie the activation of nociceptive systems which transmit both proximal and referred pain stimuli associated with MPS.

Musculoskeletal Pain Associated with Fibromyalgia

It is important to distinguish the terminologies associated with the underpinnings of musculoskeletal pain associated with fibromyalgia and contrast them with those that describe the origins of pain related to MPS. Fibromyalgia (a disorder with psychological and social components) is partially characterized by widespread musculoskeletal pain with allodynic and hyperalgesic components. While in some respects symptomatically similar to MPS, muscles of fibromyalgia patients

do not present with taut bands of hypercontracted myofibers [19]; instead, muscles throughout the body present with tender points [3, 16, 20]. There is some disagreement as to whether the appearance of tender points in muscles and the occurrence of musculoskeletal pain throughout the body are generalized events in patients suffering from fibromyalgia. Some believe that the regionally localized onset and spread of MPS is a characteristic which distinguishes it from the more generalized occurrence of tender points and musculoskeletal pain associated with fibromyalgia [16, 19, 21]. Still other evidence suggests that some forms of fibromyalgia begin with local or regional pain that later precedes widespread musculoskeletal pain [22–25]. Regardless of these points of contention, the underlying mechanisms generating the sensation of musculoskeletal pain associated with fibromyalgia likely significantly overlap with the pathways of pain perception in most muscle injury and disorder models.

Neural Mechanisms of Musculoskeletal Pain Perception

Peripheral Mechanism: The Nociceptive System

Nociceptors are peripheral afferent sensory neurons with free nerve endings located in peripheral tissue, which also make synaptic connections with ascending second-order central sensory neurons in the dorsal horn of the spinal cord. Nociceptors are either thinly myelinated (group III; Aδ-type) fibers or unmyelinated (group IV; C-type) fibers. There is ample evidence from animal studies that both group III and group IV afferent nociceptors are present and active in skeletal muscle of mammals [26, 27]. Nociceptors respond to both noxious mechanical stimuli and chemical stimuli associated with damaged tissue. Importantly, in normal physiologic conditions, nociceptors associated with skeletal muscles are not activated by normal muscle contraction or stretch, or any other nonnoxious stimulus and are thus considered high-threshold mechanosensitive. Of note, similar to sensory receptors associated with cutaneous tissue,

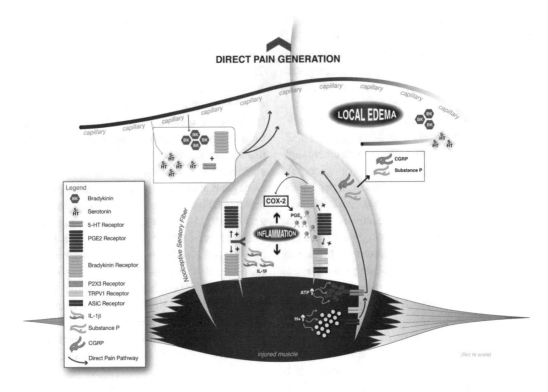

Fig. 5.1 Summary model of the humoral and local origins of musculoskeletal pain. At the onset of inflammation following muscle injury, the humoral protein bradykinin *(BK)* increasingly binds to the upregulated kinin B2 receptor expressed by nociceptive neurons, activating them. Additionally, upregulated in circulation by muscle inflammation is serotonin *(5-HT)*, which both activates nociceptive neurons and increases their sensitivity to BK. Further, sensitizing nociceptive neurons to BK is the inflammation-activated, locally synthesized lipid prostaglandin E_2 *(PGE$_2$)*. Local pain factors arise following nociceptor activation with the release of the peptides substance P *(SP)* and calcitonin gene-related peptide *(CGRP)* which serve as vasodilators to induce local edema. With the onset of edema, there is local increase in the production of the cytokine interleukin-1 beta (IL-1β) which increases PGE_2 synthesis and the receptors for both PGE_2 and BK. Other local factors influencing musculoskeletal pain are the increased concentrations of extracellular adenosine triphosphate *(ATP)* due to damaged muscle membranes following injury. ATP via activation of the P2X3 receptor can directly activate nociceptive neurons. In addition, with advancing local edema and ischemia associated with muscle damage, the pH of the local cellular environment drops, thus increasing the concentration of protons (H^+). The H^+-activated transient receptor potential cation channel subfamily V, member 1 *(TRPV1)* and the acid-sensing ion channels are stimulated by the increased H^+ concentration and directly activate muscle-associated nociceptors. (Courtesy of Elizabeth A. Drum)

nociceptors may respond to both chemical and mechanical stimuli (polymodal) or respond only to chemical or mechanical stimuli (unimodal) [28].

Muscle-associated nociceptors are classically activated by a number of humoral and cellular factors (summarized in Fig. 5.1), including the peptide bradykinin (BK) , the modified amine paracrine hormone serotonin (5-HT), the lipid prostanoid prostaglandin E_2 (PGE$_2$), and adenosine triphosphate (ATP). Additionally, locally high potassium ion (K^+) concentration activates subsets of nociceptors [6, 27, 29–31]. BK is a humoral peptide enzymatically cleaved from a precursor plasma globulin, high molecular weight (HMW) kininogen, which is synthesized in the liver. Enzymatic cleavage of HMW kininogen to form BK is mediated by the plasma protease kallikrein [32]. BK exerts it effects through the kinin B1 and B2 G-protein-coupled receptors. In homeostatic conditions, BK generally binds to the B2 receptor expressed by skeletal muscle-associated nociceptive neurons. However, during inflammatory events, the B1 receptor is upregulated in nociceptive nerve endings, and BK subsequently exerts algesic musculoskeletal effects via this G-protein-coupled receptor which is excitatory to muscle nociceptors upon activation [33–35].

Studies demonstrate that 5-HT can exert a direct and independent algesic effect when injected into skeletal muscle [36]. Importantly, if 5-HT injection precedes BK injection by only a few minutes, the resulting musculoskeletal pain is significantly increased [37–40]. Thus, 5-HT seems to act both independently as a nociceptive factor and synergistically with BK to hypersensitize nociceptors to increased local BK concentrations following muscle injury. In both human and animal studies, 5-HT injection elicits immediate muscle tenderness, but concurrent with this direct algesic effect is the seemly simultaneous hypersensitization of the muscle nociceptors to BK. Supporting this, BK administration following 5-HT injection in these studies moves skeletal muscle from a state of tenderness to a state of musculoskeletal pain when stimulated by otherwise weak, non-noxious mechanical stimuli, a hallmark of hyperalgesia associated with many muscular disorders and injuries [39–41]. BK injection alone does not elicit the same level of pain, thus supporting the hypothesis that nociceptors must undergo a hypersensitization process to generate the level of musculoskeletal pain associated with muscle damage.

In contrast to the direct effects of 5-HT on the onset of musculoskeletal pain, PGE_2 does not have any known primary algesic effects on skeletal muscle, as demonstrated by studies showing that injection of the lipid into muscles does not elicit musculoskeletal pain [36]. The role of PGE_2 in the onset of muscle pain seems to be to directly hypersensitize musculoskeletal nociceptors to BK. Supporting this idea, muscle nociceptors with a high threshold for mechanical stimuli for activation dramatically increase their sensitivity and propensity for pain generation following PGE_2 injection and subsequent BK treatment [36]. The relationship between PGE_2 and BK in the sensitization of muscle-associated nociceptors and the onset of musculoskeletal pain strongly informs

our current models and understanding of the discomfort and soreness that results from muscle damage following overload or overuse. Muscle damage leads to local inflammation and increased BK concentrations in the area of insult. Likewise, tissue damage leads to the upregulation and increased activity of cyclooxygenase-2 (COX-2), the enzyme that mediates the conversion of arachidonic acid to active PGE_2. The mechanism by which PGE_2 hypersensitizes muscle-associated nociceptors to BK is currently unknown. The two PGE_2 receptor isoforms known to be expressed by nociceptor nerve endings, EP1 (prostaglandin E receptor 1) and EP4 (prostaglandin E receptor 4), are G-protein-coupled receptors, which activate protein kinase C (PKC) and protein kinase A (PKA) pathways, respectively [42]. PGE_2-mediated hypersensitization of muscle-associated nociceptors to BK is unlikely to be immediately at the gene transcription regulatory level due to the time course of sensitization (minutes). Rather, the downstream effects of EP1 and/or EP4 activation likely modify the activity of existing B1 receptors expressed by nociceptive neurons, or possibly their affinity for the BK ligand. Supporting this line of reasoning, other known activators of nociceptors, transient receptor potential vanilloid-1 (TRPV1) channels, the purinergic P2X3 receptor, and the tetrodotoxin-resistant voltage-gated sodium (Na^+) channel $Na_v1.9$ (each discussed in detail below) are targets of EP1 and EP4 modification [43–45]. Future studies should delineate the specific mechanism by which PGE_2 hypersensitizes nociceptors to BK and whether EP1 and/or EP4 signal transduction cascades target the B1 receptor during muscle inflammation.

While PGE_2 influences the strength of BK signaling and subsequent nociceptor activation, BK and local signaling factors stored in the free endings of nociceptors regulate PGE_2 release in an area of tissue damage. Substance P (SP) and calcitonin gene-related peptide (CGRP) are neuropeptides expressed by nociceptors, but do not directly elicit pain after injection into muscle. However, activation of nociceptors induces the release of SP and CGRP from nerve endings, which go on to act as strong vasodilators and lead to local edema [46]. The induction of edema leads to further increases in both BK and PGE$_2$ release in the area of inflammation and pain generation increases significantly. As edema and inflammatory processes progress, there is a local increased release of the cytokine interleukin-1 beta (IL-1β). IL-1β signaling has been shown to increase both COX-2 and prostaglandin EP1 and EP4 expression [47, 48] as well as upregulate both kinin B1 and B2 receptor gene expression [49, 50]. Thus, a process that some have described as "a vicious cycle" [34] is induced in which signaling factors regulating pain generation and inflammation and edema also enhance each other's activity. These cyclic signaling pathways are expected to underlie the induction of musculoskeletal pain, tenderness, and possibly TrP formation associated with muscular disorders such as DOMS, fibromyalgia, and MPS, respectively. Current strategies (see inset, Fig. 5.1) to inhibit the recurrent induction of pain and edema pathways include the wide use of nonsteroidal anti-inflammatory drugs (NSAIDS) that specifically inhibit the activity of COX-1 and COX-2 enzymes, thereby reducing prostaglandin signaling. Another promising drug currently under investigation is fasitibant chloride, a selective kinin B2 receptor antagonist. In animal studies, fasitibant chloride has been shown to inhibit the synergistic activity of BK and IL-1β to increase COX-2 gene expression and PGE$_2$ release [51] and serves to significantly reduce inflammatory events [52].

As mentioned earlier, nociceptors are activated by a number of intra- and extracellular signaling molecules. The metabolically important nucleoside triphosphate ATP can bind to the membrane purinergic receptor P2X3 and induce excitatory Na$^+$ currents in nociceptive neurons [53, 54]. Muscle membrane damage due to overload, overuse, or pathological processes leads to ATP diffusion from the myofiber cytoplasm into the extracellular environment. Subsequent activation of P2X3 receptors by ATP is sufficient to induce excitation in muscle-associated group IV afferent nociceptors which leads to pain generation [55, 56]. This mechanism is highly associated with muscle damage due to overload or overuse, as well as injury occurring from eccentric muscle contraction. Other novel activators of

nociceptor are the proton (H$^+$)-sensitive TRPV1 channels and acid-sensing ion channels (ASICs). These channels are activated by increased H$^+$ ion concentration or lowered pH [57]. Importantly, lowered pH in muscle tissue is associated with a number of conditions, including overwork, inflammatory processes, and muscular ischemia. A lowered pH of 6.0 is sufficient to activate both TRPV1 and ASICs and subsequently excite musculoskeletal nociceptors [31]. In animal studies, antagonists to P2X3 receptors, TRPV1 channels, and ASICs were able to reverse hyperalgesia processes associated with DOMS following eccentric muscle contractions indicating the significant role these excitatory ion channels play in musculoskeletal pain generation [58]. Also of importance, profound muscular ischemia is associated with the taut bands of the TrPs found in MPS patients [59]. Likewise, reduced blood flow to skeletal muscle has been described as common symptom among those suffering from fibromyalgia [60]. These findings may indicate that a lowered pH and activation of TRPV1 channels and ASICs expressed by musculoskeletal nociceptors may contribute to pain associated with these disorders.

Central Mechanism: Dorsal Spinal Cord and Brain Stem

Axonal projections from musculoskeletal nociceptive neurons enter the dorsal root ganglia to provide input to the dorsal horn of the spinal cord and to the trigeminal nucleus pars caudalis of the brain stem (see Fig. 5.2). The sensory dorsal horn of the spinal cord is divided into five laminae, of which laminae III, IV, V, and a small division of lamina II are innervated mainly by hair follicle and tactile sensory Aδ- and Aβ-fibers. The primary nociceptive group III (Aδ-fibers; lightly myelinated) and group IV (C-fibers; unmyelinated) afferents innervating skeletal muscle terminate in dorsal horn lamina I and a large portion of lamina II [61]. Group IV nociceptive neurons are classified as being peptidergic (expressing SP and CGRP) or non-peptidergic [62, 63]. Peptidergic nociceptive group IV afferents include those

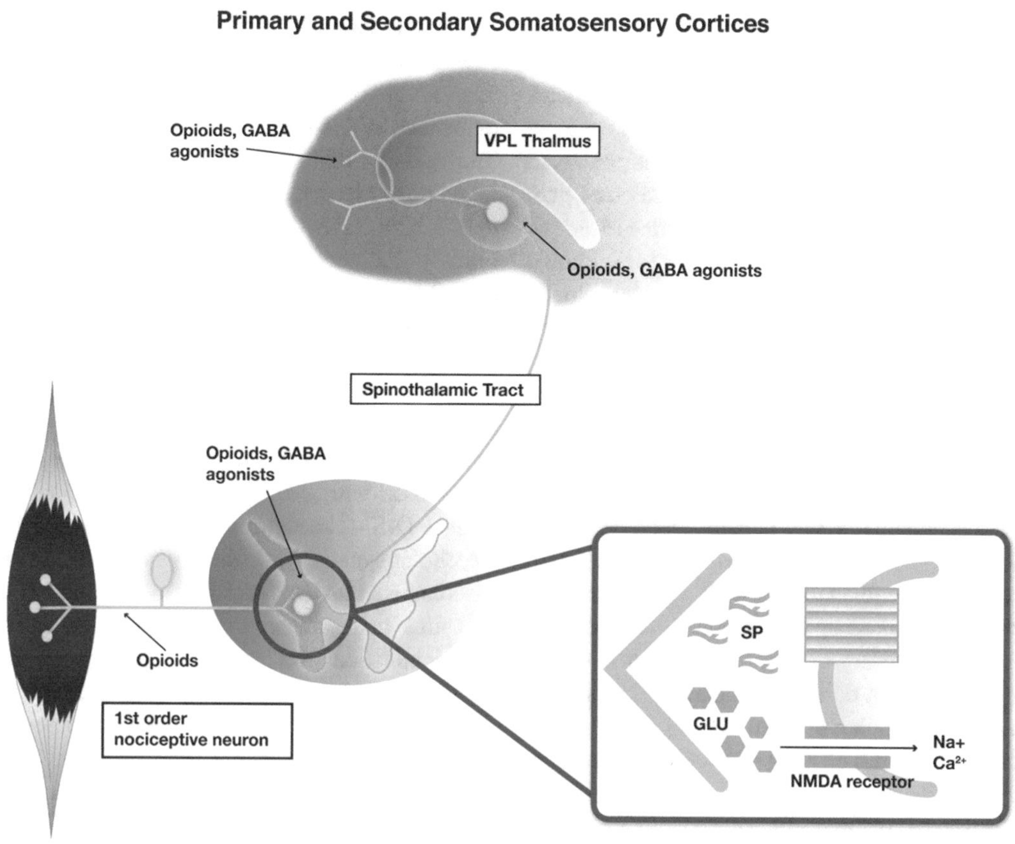

Primary and Secondary Somatosensory Cortices

Fig. 5.2 Central pain-processing pathways and pharmaceutical analgesic targets. To date, the most often prescribed central treatments for musculoskeletal pain target inhibitory γ-amino butyric acid *(GABA)*-ergic interneurons, using GABAergic or opioid receptor agonists, throughout the neural pain-processing pathway from first-order nociceptive neurons in the periphery to second-order neurons in the spinal cord, to third- and fourth-order neurons in the thalamus and cortex. (Courtesy of Elizabeth A. Drum)

associated with musculoskeletal tissue, while non-peptidergic afferents generally consist of sensory neurons with nerve endings in the epidermis [64, 65]. The primary neurotransmitter utilized by all nociceptive afferent neurons is the excitatory amino acid glutamate, although SP and CGRP are common neuropeptide co-transmitters [62]. Primary afferent nociceptors make excitatory synapses with second-order neurons in the dorsal horn, which, in turn, ascend in the lateral spinothalamic tract to target the ventral posterior lateral (VPL) and ventral posterior medial (VPM) nuclei of the thalamus. Tertiary sensory neurons of the VPL and VPM carry nociceptive information to the primary and secondary somatosensory cortices [61].

Many of the neural mechanisms that regulate the central processing of pain information remain largely uncharacterized. Among the better understood phenomena associated with central pain relays is the neurophysiology underlying the occurrences of referred pain and secondary hyperalgesia and allodynia. Fundamental to these types of pain perception is the widespread collateral synapses made by group III and group IV nociceptive afferent neurons as they innervate laminae I and II of the of the dorsal horn of the spinal cord [66]. These branching axons from primary nociceptive neurons create overlapping receptive fields and the potential for the creation of new receptive fields. As an example of referred pain in humans, the secondary sensory neurons of lamina

I of the dorsal horn receive nociceptor innervation from musculature of the shoulder, while also receiving nociceptor afferents from the pericardium of the heart. If the pericardial nociceptors become significantly active, the pain is perceived in the shoulder [67]. Expansion of referred pain may be due to the development of new receptive fields in the dorsal spinal cord in process known as central sensitization. The neurons of the dorsal spinal cord display remarkable plasticity in their receptive fields as demonstrated in animal studies in which BK was injected into the tibialis anterior muscle of rats. In a short time, dorsal horn neural representation of the injected muscle had expanded to include the area also representing the biceps femoris muscle [68]. There is a time-dependent component of referred pain generation in humans in which there is a 20–40 s interval between the immediate perception of localized pain and the secondary onset of referred pain [69]. It is assumed that during this delay, neural signaling of overlapping afferent nociceptive fibers in the dorsal horn is creating new receptive fields by activating previously silent synapses.

In the case of hyperalgesia and allodynia, prolonged and intense noxious activation of musculoskeletal nociceptors triggers the strengthening and expansion of existing synapses. The currently accepted model of secondary hyperalgesia is homosynaptic and represents a significant potentiation of the synapses formed between the peripheral nociceptors and dorsal horn neurons, such that a greater postsynaptic response is elicited from a noxious stimulus [67]. Allodynia is understood to involve a heterosynaptic process coupling non-nociceptive peripheral sensory afferent signaling to nociceptive afferent activity. For example, group I (Aβ) sensory afferents normally are activated by non-noxious mechanical stimuli, and while active during a singular noxious stimulus, will not normally excite the neurons of the spinothalamic tract. However, protracted, intense group IV nociceptive signaling to the dorsal spinal cord can lead to the potentiation of non-nociceptive synapses and activation of spinothalamic neurons, such that a previously non-noxious stimulus will be perceived as painful [67].

Another clinically relevant concept regarding central nociception processing is the transition from a state of acute pain to chronic pain that is associated with a number of muscular disorders. The basis of this phenomenon is the plasticity inherent to afferent nociceptive synapses in the dorsal horn. Glutamate released by nociceptors binds to the postsynaptic N-methyl-D-aspartate (NMDA) receptors which allow for an influx of Ca^{2+} which drives the activation of a host of signal-transduction cascades. Sustained NMDA receptor activation leads to the insertion of new receptors, expansion of the synaptic area, and overall potentiation of the synapse. Likewise, SP, co-released with glutamate, binds to the neurokinin-1 (NK-1) receptor and induces several intracellular synaptic potentiating pathways. Pharmacological blockade of both NMDA and NK-1 receptors using antagonists delivered by intrathecal injection prevents secondary hyperalgesia and receptive field expansion in nociceptive dorsal horn neurons [70]. Prolonged activation of dorsal horn neurons by nociceptor afferent neurons leads to abnormally potentiated synapses. Progressing toward a state of chronic pain, research demonstrates that with prolonged overactivity, nociceptor afferents begin to sprout new axon terminals and form synapses with novel dorsal horn sensory neurons, which ultimately serves to expand their receptive field. In addition to the hypersensitization of dorsal horn neurons and an expansion of their receptive fields, overactivity of glutamatergic/SP synapses may also lead to excitotoxicity and cell death in some neural populations. In particular, the inhibitory γ-amino butyric acid (GABA) interneurons of the dorsal horn are very susceptible to overexcitation [71]. When tonically activated, NMDA/SP receptor-mediated Ca^{2+} influx can trigger the activation of intracellular mechanisms that lead to apoptotic death. GABAergic interneurons of the dorsal spinal cord serve to inhibit overactivity of second-order nociceptive neurons. In this model of chronic pain onset, the result of prolonged, intense musculoskeletal pain is the appearance of populations of hyperactive, potentiated second-order nociceptive neurons with expanded receptive fields, which are no longer inhibited by

GABAergic interneurons [31]. This series of cellular events may bring about much of the chronic pain experienced by sufferers of fibromyalgia and similar disorder disorders.

Conclusions

A clear understanding of the peripheral and central mechanisms that give rise to the experience of acute and chronic musculoskeletal pain is critical for the evaluation and treatment of individuals experiencing musculoskeletal pain. This knowledge provides a conceptual framework that helps clinicians make distinctions between acute and chronic disorders. Appreciation of these differences and the potential for simultaneous or overlapping etiologies of musculoskeletal pain should inform treatment recommendations and improve outcomes in these debilitating disorders. In addition, the understanding that musculoskeletal pain origins are often distinct from other nociceptive pathways is an important concept in future strategies to identify and treat pain arising from musculoskeletal origins. From targeting peripheral nociceptive factors to limiting the activity of central sensitizing pathways, future research should focus on both improving treatment for acute pain and preventative treatments that will halt the "vicious cycle" before hyperalgesia or chronic pain become inevitable.

References

1. Crow WT, Willis DR. Estimating cost of care for patients with acute low back pain: a retrospective review of patient records. J Am Osteopath Assoc. 2009;109(4):229–33.
2. Picavet HS, Hazes JM. Prevalence of self reported musculoskeletal diseases is high. Ann Rheum Dis. 2003;62(7):644–50.
3. Woolf AD, et al. Musculoskeletal pain in Europe: its impact and a comparison of population and medical perceptions of treatment in eight European countries. Ann Rheum Dis. 2004;63(4):342–7.
4. Krismer M, van Tulder M. Strategies for prevention and management of musculoskeletal conditions. Low back pain (non-specific). Best Pract Res Clin Rheumatol. 2007;21(1):77–91.
5. Drewes AM, Jennum P. Epidemiology of myofascial pain, low back pain, morning stiffness and sleep-related complaints in the general population. J Musculoskelet Pain. 1995;3(1):121.
6. Mense S. Muscle pain: mechanisms and clinical significance. Dtsch Arztebl Int. 2008;105(12):214–9.
7. Kellgren JH. Referred pains from muscle. Br Med J. 1938;1(4023):325–7.
8. Mense S, Simons DG. Muscle pain: understanding its nature, diagnosis, and treatment. Baltimore: Lippincott Williams, & Wilkins; 2001.
9. Hockaday JM, Whitty CW. Patterns of referred pain in the normal subject. Brain. 1967;90(3):481–96.
10. Herren-Gerber R, et al. Modulation of central hypersensitivity by nociceptive input in chronic pain after whiplash injury. Pain Med. 2004;5(4):366–76.
11. Fernandez-de-Las-Penas C, et al. The local and referred pain from myofascial trigger points in the temporalis muscle contributes to pain profile in chronic tension-type headache. Clin J Pain. 2007;23(9):786–92.
12. Arendt-Nielsen L, Graven-Nielsen T. Translational musculoskeletal pain research. Best Pract Res Clin Rheumatol. 2011;25(2):209–26.
13. Wheeler AH, Aaron GW. Muscle pain due to injury. Curr Pain Headache Rep. 2001;5(5):441–6.
14. Lewis PB, Ruby D, Bush-Joseph CA. Muscle soreness and delayed-onset muscle soreness. Clin Sports Med. 2012;31(2):255–62.
15. Simons DG. Review of enigmatic MTrPs as a common cause of enigmatic musculoskeletal pain and dysfunction. J Electromyogr Kinesiol. 2004;14(1):95–107.
16. Gerwin RD. Classification epidemiology and natural history of myofascial pain syndrome. Curr Pain Headache Rep. 2001;5(5):412–20.
17. Scott NA, et al. Trigger point injections for chronic non-malignant musculoskeletal pain: a systematic review. Pain Med. 2009;10(1):54–69.
18. Giamberardino MA, et al. Myofascial pain syndromes and their evaluation. Best Pract Res Clin Rheumatol. 2011;25(2):185–98.
19. Rau C-L, Russell IJ. Regional versus generalized muscle pain syndromes. Curr Rev Pain. 1999;3:85–95.
20. Wolfe F, et al. The American College of Rheumatology 1990 criteria for the classification of fibromyalgia. Report of the multicenter criteria committee. Arthritis Rheum. 1990;33(2):160–72.
21. Rau CL, Russell IJ. Is fibromyalgia a distinct clinical syndrome? Curr Rev Pain. 2000;4(4):287–94.
22. Delorme T, et al. Clinical study of chronic pain in hereditary myopathies. Eur J Pain. 2004;8(1):55–61.
23. Kosek E, Ordeberg G. Abnormalities of somatosensory perception in patients with painful osteoarthritis normalize following successful treatment. Eur J Pain. 2000;4(3):229–38.
24. Leffler AS, et al. Somatosensory perception and function of diffuse noxious inhibitory controls (DNIC) in patients suffering from rheumatoid arthritis. Eur J Pain. 2002;6(2):161–76.

25. Nielsen LA, Henriksson KG. Pathophysiological mechanisms in chronic musculoskeletal pain (fibromyalgia): the role of central and peripheral sensitization and pain disinhibition. Best Pract Res Clin Rheumatol. 2007;21(3):465–80.

26. Diehl B, Hoheisel U, Mense S. The influence of mechanical stimuli and of acetylsalicylic acid on the discharges of slowly conducting afferent units from normal and inflamed muscle in the rat. Exp Brain Res. 1993;92(3):431–40.

27. Mense S, Meyer H. Different types of slowly conducting afferent units in cat skeletal muscle and tendon. J Physiol. 1985;363:403–17.

28. Millan MJ. The induction of pain: an integrative review. Prog Neurobiol. 1999;57(1):1–164.

29. Kumazawa T, Mizumura K. Thin-fibre receptors responding to mechanical, chemical, and thermal stimulation in the skeletal muscle of the dog. J Physiol. 1977;273(1):179–94.

30. Kaufman MP, et al. Effects of capsaicin and bradykinin on afferent fibers with ending in skeletal muscle. Circ Res. 1982;50(1):133–9.

31. Mense S. The pathogenesis of muscle pain. Curr Pain Headache Rep. 2003;7(6):419–25.

32. Bjorkqvist J, Jamsa A, Renne T. Plasma kallikrein: the bradykinin-producing enzyme. Thromb Haemost. 2013;110(3):399–407.

33. Dray A. Kinins and their receptors in hyperalgesia. Can J Physiol Pharmacol. 1997;75(6):704–12.

34. Graven-Nielsen T, Mense S. The peripheral apparatus of muscle pain: evidence from animal and human studies. Clin J Pain. 2001;17(1):2–10.

35. Perkins MN, Kelly D. Induction of bradykinin B1 receptors in vivo in a model of ultra-violet irradiation-induced thermal hyperalgesia in the rat. Br J Pharmacol. 1993;110(4):1441–4.

36. Mense S. Sensitization of group IV muscle receptors to bradykinin by 5-hydroxytryptamine and prostaglandin E2. Brain Res. 1981;225(1):95–105.

37. Jensen K, et al. Pain, wheal and flare in human forearm skin induced by bradykinin and 5-hydroxytryptamine. Peptides. 1990;11(6):1133–8.

38. Jensen K, et al. Pain and tenderness in human temporal muscle induced by bradykinin and 5-hydroxytryptamine. Peptides. 1990;11(6):1127–32.

39. Babenko VV, et al. Experimental human muscle pain induced by intramuscular injections of bradykinin, serotonin, and substance P. Eur J Pain. 1999;3(2):93–102.

40. Babenko V, et al. Experimental human muscle pain and muscular hyperalgesia induced by combinations of serotonin and bradykinin. Pain. 1999;82(1):1–8.

41. Babenko V, et al. Duration and distribution of experimental muscle hyperalgesia in humans following combined infusions of serotonin and bradykinin. Brain Res. 2000;853(2):275–81.

42. Kawabata A. Prostaglandin E2 and pain–an update. Biol Pharm Bull. 2011;34(8):1170–3.

43. Villarreal CF, et al. The role of Na(V)1.8 sodium channel in the maintenance of chronic inflammatory hypernociception. Neurosci Lett. 2005;386(2):72–7.

44. Wang C, Li GW, Huang LY. Prostaglandin E2 potentiation of P2X3 receptor mediated currents in dorsal root ganglion neurons. Mol Pain. 2007;3:22.

45. Moriyama T, et al. Sensitization of TRPV1 by EP1 and IP reveals peripheral nociceptive mechanism of prostaglandins. Mol Pain. 2005;1:3.

46. Pedersen-Bjergaard U, et al. Calcitonin gene-related peptide, neurokinin A and substance P: effects on nociception and neurogenic inflammation in human skin and temporal muscle. Peptides. 1991;12(2):333–7.

47. Alvarez-Soria MA, et al. Prostaglandin E2 receptors EP1 and EP4 are up-regulated in rabbit chondrocytes by IL-1beta, but not by TNFalpha. Rheumatol Int. 2007;27(10):911–7.

48. Angel J, et al. Interleukin-1-induced prostaglandin E2 biosynthesis in human synovial cells involves the activation of cytosolic phospholipase A2 and cyclo-oxygenase-2. Eur J Biochem. 1994;226(1):125–31.

49. Murakami M, Ohta T, Ito S. Interleukin-1beta enhances the action of bradykinin in rat myenteric neurons through up-regulation of glial B1 receptor expression. Neuroscience. 2008;151(1):222–31.

50. Schmidlin F, et al. Interleukin-1beta induces bradykinin B2 receptor gene expression through a prostanoid cyclic AMP-dependent pathway in human bronchial smooth muscle cells. Mol Pharmacol. 1998;53(6):1009–15.

51. Meini S, et al. Fasitibant prevents the bradykinin and interleukin 1beta synergism on prostaglandin E(2) release and cyclooxygenase 2 expression in human fibroblast-like synoviocytes. Naunyn Schmiedebergs Arch Pharmacol. 2012;385(8):777–86.

52. Valenti C, et al. Fasitibant chloride, a kinin B(2) receptor antagonist, and dexamethasone interact to inhibit carrageenan-induced inflammatory arthritis in rats. Br J Pharmacol. 2012;166(4):1403–10.

53. Burnstock G. P2X receptors in sensory neurones. Br J Anaesth. 2000;84(4):476–88.

54. Ding Y, et al. ATP, P2X receptors and pain pathways. J Auton Nerv Syst. 2000;81(1–3):289–94.

55. Hamilton SG, McMahon SB. ATP as a peripheral mediator of pain. J Auton Nerv Syst. 2000;81(1–3):187–94.

56. Cook SP, McCleskey EW. Cell damage excites nociceptors through release of cytosolic ATP. Pain. 2002;95(1–2):41–7.

57. McCleskey EW, Gold MS. Ion channels of nociception. Annu Rev Physiol. 1999;61:835–56.

58. Fujii Y, et al. TRP channels and ASICs mediate mechanical hyperalgesia in models of inflammatory muscle pain and delayed onset muscle soreness. Pain. 2008;140(2):292–304.

59. Bruckle W, et al. Tissue pO2 measurement in taut back musculature (m. erector spinae). Z Rheumatol. 1990;49(4):208–16.

60. Staud R. Future perspectives: pathogenesis of chronic muscle pain. Best Pract Res Clin Rheumatol. 2007;21(3):581–96.

61. Todd AJ. Neuronal circuitry for pain processing in the dorsal horn. Nat Rev Neurosci. 2010;11(12):823–36.

62. Lawson SN, Crepps BA, Perl ER. Relationship of substance P to afferent characteristics of dorsal root ganglion neurones in guinea-pig. J Physiol. 1997;505(Pt 1):177–91.
63. Snider WD, McMahon SB. Tackling pain at the source: new ideas about nociceptors. Neuron. 1998;20(4):629–32.
64. Taylor AM, Peleshok JC, Ribeiro-da-Silva A. Distribution of P2X(3)-immunoreactive fibers in hairy and glabrous skin of the rat. J Comp Neurol. 2009;514(6):555–66.
65. Bennett DL, et al. trkA, CGRP and IB4 expression in retrogradely labelled cutaneous and visceral primary sensory neurones in the rat. Neurosci Lett. 1996;206(1):33–6.
66. Perl ER, Kruger L. Nociception and pain: evolution of concepts and observations in touch and pain. In: Kruger L, editor. New York: Academic; 1996. p. 180–212.
67. Lewin GR, Moshourab R. Mechanosensation and pain. J Neurobiol. 2004;61(1):30–44.
68. Mense S. Referral of muscle pain. New aspects. Ame Pain Soc J. 1994;3:1–9.
69. Gibson W, Arendt-Nielsen L, Graven-Nielsen T. Referred pain and hyperalgesia in human tendon and muscle belly tissue. Pain. 2006;120(1–2):113–23.
70. Hoheisel U, Sander B, Mense S. Myositis-induced functional reorganisation of the rat dorsal horn: effects of spinal superfusion with antagonists to neurokinin and glutamate receptors. Pain. 1997;69(3):219–30.
71. Yezierski RP, et al. Excitotoxic spinal cord injury: behavioral and morphological characteristics of a central pain model. Pain. 1998;75(1):141–55.

Part II
Assessment of Muscular Injuries in the Posterior Leg

Clinical Assessment of the Posterior Leg

6

J. Bryan Dixon and Christopher Robert Faber

Introduction

Leg pain is one of the most common presenting patient complaints and is attributable to almost 8 million physician office visits a year. Only pain in the spine, shoulder, and knee are more common musculoskeletal-related complaints [1]. Although the focus of this book is on muscular injuries, posterior leg pain can arise from a variety of causes (Fig. 6.1). Health-care professionals conducting the initial evaluation of leg pain are faced with the difficult challenge of sorting through a diverse differential of orthopedic, neurologic, rheumatologic, and vascular etiologies to arrive at the correct diagnosis. Fortunately, the history and physical exam are quite helpful in determining the root cause of posterior leg pain.

The goal of this chapter is to provide a functional and practical guide to the physical examination of the posterior leg. The level and scope of the material presented is intended to be inclusive of the needs of a variety of health-care profes-

sionals. In general, physicians need to have a broader scope with an eye towards referred pain or signs of systemic medical problems while rehabilitation professionals require a more detailed working knowledge of musculoskeletal etiologies for pain and dysfunction. The chapter is organized into sections covering the standard examination areas: inspection, gait and station, palpation, range of motion (ROM), strength testing, neurologic status, vascular status, and special tests. An attempt has been made to correlate exam finding with the associated diagnosis in the differential.

Acute injuries often necessitate a more circumscribed examination due to pain and more limited goals of determining the specifics of the injury location and severity. In acute injuries, it is also important to evaluate for potential complications and be cognizant of confounding or coexisting injuries. For chronic or sub-acute complaints, a more comprehensive and functional approach is required. Particular attention should be paid to predisposing factors for injury and referred pain from neurologic, vascular, and bony pathology. There is some wisdom in the playful joke that the only aptitude needed to do orthopedics is the capability to compare one side of the body to the other. So whenever possible, take advantage of the natural symmetry of the body to compare apparent abnormal finding relative to the contralateral limb.

J. B. Dixon (✉)
Sports Medicine, Advanced Center for Orthopedics, Marquette, MI, USA
e-mail: jbryandixon@hotmail.com

C. R. Faber
Emergency Department, Baraga County Memorial Hospital, L'Anse, MI, USA
e-mail: chrisfaber77@gmail.com

Musculoskeletal
Muscle Strains/Ruptures*
Gastrocnemius*
Soleus*
Plantaris
Popliteus
Tibialis Posterior
Flexor Hallux Longus
Flexor Digitorum Longus
Tendinopathy*
Achilles*
Posterior Tibialis*
Flexor Hallucis Longus
Proximal Gastrocnemius
Distal Biceps Femoris
Popliteus
Contusions*
Gastrocnemius*
Periosteal
Stress Fractures*
Fibula*
Posterior Cortex of the Tibia *
Acute fractures
Tibia
Fibula
Maisonneuve fracture
Tibial Periostitis*
Muscle Herniations
Baker's Cysts*
Ganglion Cysts
Posterior Cruciate Ligament Strain
Posterior Knee Capsular Sprain
Per Anserine Bursitis
Accessory Soleus
Referred Pain from Proximal Tibiofibular Joint
Subluxation
Osteoarthritis
Ganglion Cyst
Delayed Onset Muscle Soreness*
Rhabdomyolysis
Tibiofibular Syndesmosis Injuries
Knee Joint Effusion *
Bone Tumors
Osteosarcoma
Osteoid Osteoma
Bilobular Calcifying Fibrous Pseudotumor
*Indicates Common Causes Of Posterior Leg Symptoms

Vascular
Chronic Compartment Syndrome*
Deep Posterior*

Fig. 6.1 Differential diagnosis of posterior leg pain, weakness, or swelling

Superficial Posterior
Vascular Insufficiency/Claudication*
Atherosclerotic Disease*
Deep Venous Thrombosis*
Varicose Veins*
Superficial Thrombophlebitis*
Post-Thrombotic Syndrome
Popliteal Artery Entrapment
Acute Arterial Occlusion
Acute Compartment Syndrome
Endofibrosis Of External Iliac Artery
Femoral Endarteritis
Diabetic Muscle Infraction
Intramuscular Hemangioma

*Indicates Common Causes Of Posterior Leg Symptoms

Neurologic
Lumbar Radiculopathy*
Lumbosacral Plexopathy
Lower Extremity Mononeuropathy
Sciatic
Femoral
Saphenous
Fibular (Peroneal) Nerve Injury
Superficial Peroneal Nerve Entrapment
Tibial Nerve Injury
Compression In Popliteal Fossa
Tarsal Tunnel Syndrome With Proximal Radiation
Complex Regional Pain Syndrome Type 1
Polyneuropathy
Referred Pain From Myofascial Structures
Neuroma

*Indicates Common Causes Of Posterior Leg Symptoms

Rheumatologic, Metabolic and Inflammatory
Electrolyte and Metabolic Disturbances
Muscle Cramping*
Sickle Cell Trait
Rickets
Paget's Disease Of Bone
Muscular Dystrophy and Congenital Myopathies
Polymyositis
Hemochromatosis
Myositis Ossificans
Hyperparathyroidism
Hypothyroidism
Sarcoidosis
Erythema Nodosum
Crystalline Disease
Spondyloarthropathies and Enthesopathies

Fig. 6.1 (continued)

| Fibromyalgia/Myofascial Pain Syndrome |
| Osteomyelitis |
| Cellulitis * |
| Bacterial Myositis |
| Abscess |
| Statin Medications |

*Indicates Common Cause of Posterior Leg Symptoms

Fig. 6.1 (continued)

Inspection

It is important to completely visualize the bilateral lower extremities during the examination. This is best accomplished by having the patient disrobe or change into examination shorts prior to beginning the evaluation. During inspection careful attention should be paid to signs of bruising, swelling, and skin changes that may suggest underlying vascular or neurologic disease. Visible erythema and swelling associated with pain and increased warmth are the classic signs of inflammation and should prompt the clinician to consider inflammatory causes of leg pain. Inflammatory causes of leg pain can be localized or systemic. Leg pain in the presence of skin rashes and nail abnormalities are also suggestive of possible systemic inflammatory conditions. Scars or wounds on the legs should be noted and correlated with the past medical and surgical history.

If bruising is found, note the location, size, distribution, and color. Location and distribution of ecchymosis can suggest the location of the injury and its depth. The color of the bruising suggests the acuity of the bleeding. Upon extravasation of blood, hemoglobin begins to degrade in a sequential fashion, giving rise to progressive change in color and eventual resolution of bruising by 2 weeks. In this way, the color of the bruise can be used to age the injury: red-blue color (0–5 days), green color (5–7 days), yellow color (7–10 days), and golden-brown color (10–14 days). It should be noted that bruising or contusion refers to subcutaneous bleeding that has a traumatic etiology. Ecchymosis is a more general description of subcutaneous bleeding greater than 1 cm and may not be traumatic in etiology. Nontraumatic causes of ecchymosis include coagulopathies.

Subcutaneous bleeding less than 1 cm in diameter is either called petechia (<3 mm) or purpura (3 mm–1 cm), which are associated with platelet disorders or vasculitis, respectively. Bruising is easier to identify in patients with light skin complexions. It is common for the blood to travel along soft tissue planes which often results in migration of the bruising over time.

If calf swelling is present, take note if the calf swelling is unilateral or bilateral. Unilateral calf swelling is indicative of localized pathology whereas symmetrical swelling suggests a systemic cause. Inspection can also help determine if the swelling can be classified as pitting or non-pitting edema. Indentations from socks, shoes, or other tight-fitting clothing can be useful in detecting pitting edema. Non-pitting edema is caused by lymphedema. Pitting edema has a variety of local and systemic causes. Acute unilateral pitting edema of the leg is often due to deep venous thrombosis (DVT), cellulitis, a ruptured bakers cyst, or trauma.

Stigmata of chronic vascular disease should also be sought on inspection. Arterial peripheral vascular disease should be suspected if there are well-demarcated ulcers or non-healing lesions in the distal extremity along the ground contact areas, erythema of the foot in a dependent position which changes to pallor with elevation, and skin that is shiny, dry, and atrophic with absence of hair. Chronic venous disease is suspected on inspection if chronic soft, pitting edema is seen in the ankle and evidence of dependent varicosities of the leg with hyperpigmented skin and venous ulcerations over medial malleolus.

Inspection of the legs may also reveal stigmata of neuropathy. Thin ankles and legs along with deformities of the arch and toes can suggest hereditary neuropathies such as Charcot–Marie–Tooth (CMT) disease. Complex regional pain syndrome type 1 is associated with visible swelling and discoloration of the affected leg.

Screening for leg length should be done on inspection. A reasonable screening test of leg length symmetry can be done by observing the patient from behind while comparing the relative height of popliteal and gluteal creases. If you suspect a clinical relevant difference in leg length, additional clinical tests should be performed for further assessment. Specific examination techniques for leg length are discussed below.

Observation of the lower extremities during functional movement is important. At a minimum, inspection should be done on standing and walking. In addition, observation while running or other relevant movements can greatly aid the clinical evaluation. Evaluation of gait and station are covered separately in the next section.

Evaluation of Gait and Station

Examination of gait and station should be incorporated with the examination of the lower extremity. Because of the functional role the muscles of the posterior leg have in standing and ambulating, injuries to these muscles are often most noticeable during the evaluation of gait and station. Correlating abnormalities in gait and station to the underlying pathology requires an understanding of the normal and abnormal presentation. It should be noted that abnormities of gait and station not only can be the result of pathology but also can be causative factor in precipitating the injury. Therefore, although evaluation of gait and station can help the clinician in the diagnosis of acute muscle injuries in the posterior leg, the detailed evaluation of gait is most helpful in investigating chronic or recurrent issues that may be caused by underlying biomechanical abnormalities.

Station or stance position is evaluated by observation of the standing patient. Normal station should reveal a balanced body posture over the center of gravity and symmetrical alignment of the lower limbs and feet. In neutral stance position, alignment of the lower limb should reveal a weight-bearing line in a sagittal plane through the anterior superior iliac spine, patella, and second metatarsal of each lower extremity. The heel should be perpendicular to the forefoot and in line with the tibia. The knee should be fully extended with slight valgus alignment. The subtalar joint and hips should be in a neutral position. The pelvis should exhibit a slight anterior tilt. Significant deviations from ideal stance position suggest structural abnormalities or compensations that may lead the clinician to the diagnosis or suggest the cause of the presenting complaint (Table 6.1). When these common clinical associations are

Table 6.1 Biomechanical abnormalities commonly associated with posterior leg injury

Biomechanical abnormality	Posterior leg injury
Excessive pronation (dynamic pes planus)	Achilles tendinopathy
	Medial tibial stress syndrome
	Tibial stress fracture
	Fibular stress facture
	Tibialis posterior injury
	Flexor hallucis longus injury
Excessive supination (pes cavus)	Tibia stress fracture
	Fibular stress fracture
Hindfoot varus	Medial shin pain
	Fibular stress facture
Ankle equinus (restricted ankle dorsiflexion)	Achilles tendinopathy
	Medial tibial stress syndrome
	Calf strain
	Stress fractures

subject to evaluation by evidence-based methods the conclusions reached have been very limited [2, 3].

Gait is classically described by its two component actions called the stance phase and the swing phase. The stance phase refers to the portion of gait when the foot is on the ground, while the swing phase refers to the portion of gait when the foot is no longer in contact with the ground. The repeated progression of stance phase through swing phase produces the motion of walking and running called the gait cycle. The phases of gait are further divided into component actions. The stance phase is subdivided into heel strike, mid-stance, and push-off. The swing phase is subdivided into acceleration, mid-swing, and deceleration.

The phases of running and walking are similar. Running is defined by the addition of a flight phase between stance phases in which neither foot is in contact with the ground. While walking, 60 % of the gait cycle is spent in stance phase and 40 % in swing phase. During running, the portion of time spent in stance phase decreases with increasing running speed. In addition, running is associated with greater ROM of the pelvis, hip, and knee as well as a narrower base of gait when compared to walking.

Examination of gait can begin even before the formal exam. Observation of the patient as they ambulate through the office is most likely to reveal natural movement patterns and can quickly identify an obvious limp or the use of assistive devices. During formal examination of gait, try to identify which phase of gait and component motion is pathologic. Most abnormalities will be present in stance phase where the extremity is susceptible to the liabilities of weight bearing. Patients with muscle weakness in the gastrocnemius, soleus, and flexor hallucis longus or Achilles rupture may exhibit a flat foot gait with no or limited push-off. Gastrocnemius strains may result in the patient adopting a gait characterized by excessive knee flexion and ankle plantar flexion in an attempt to splint the affected muscle. A bouncy gait suggests early heel lift from ankle equinus or heel pain. Compensations related to ankle equinus lead to posterior leg muscles

strains, Achilles tendon injuries, shin splints, and stress fractures. Patients with fractures or other severe acute trauma will have pain in all phases of gait and are likely to either not bear weight on the affected extremity or spend as little time as possible in stance phase.

During mid-stance, as the body passes over the weight-bearing limb, the pelvis and trunk shift laterally over the weight-bearing side and drop slightly on the non-weight-bearing limb. Excessive lateral displacement during mid-stance is caused by gluteus medius weakness and results in a gluteus medius or abductor lurch gait. The Trendelenburg test evaluates the function of the gluteus medius in maintaining dynamic pelvic stability in single-leg, weight-bearing stance. The test is performed by observing the patient from behind while they are standing in double-leg stance and then in single-leg stance alternating between each leg. A positive test occurs when the pelvis does not elevate on the unsupported side during single-leg, weight bearing stance. A positive test indicates inadequate force is being generated by the gluteus medius on the stance leg to maintain dynamic pelvic stability during single-leg, weight bearing stance. This can lead to biomechanical abnormalities which increase likelihood of injuries. Inadequate gluteus medius force generation can be caused by poor gluteus medius development, poor activation sequence, nerve root mediated weakness, and anatomical variations that functionally shorten the muscle.

Excessive subtalar pronation can lead to overload of the soleus, gastrocnemius, and tibialis posterior during dynamic supination and plantar flexion. This can lead to excessive muscle tightness and soreness. In addition, overload from excessive subtalar pronation can predispose the muscles of the posterior leg to strain and tendon damage. Moreover, excessive muscle overload can cause muscular hypertrophy that can contribute to the development of compartment syndrome.

Excessive supination of the subtalar joint suggests contracture of the gastrocnemius, soleus, and tibialis posterior, structural abnormalities of the foot or weak peroneals. Excessive supination limits mobility of the foot resulting in reduced ability to attenuate force during the gait cycle and increased risk for stress fractures of the leg and foot.

Palpation

Bony Palpation

Palpation of the bones of the posterior leg is limited due to the predominance of soft tissue structures. However, palpation of bones remains an important part of the clinical examination of the posterior leg, and palpation of relevant bony landmarks of the knee and ankle is also significant. Examination by palpation is best performed with the patient seated on the edge of the examination table. This reduces the muscular tone of the leg muscles and allows the knee and ankle to be manipulated for optimal visualization and palpation of the bony landmarks. If the patient cannot sit, then it is best to position the patient supine with the knee flexed to 90°.

On the medial aspect of the leg, the tibia should be palpated along its length. Begin at the medial joint line to assess for medial joint line tenderness which can suggest osteoarthritis, medical meniscus pathology, and medial collateral ligament (MCL) strain or bursitis. Follow the medial tibia plateau distally to the distal medial collateral ligament and pes anserine insertion, then down along the medial tibia border to the medial malleolus. Focal pain along the medial tibial border can be indicative of stress fracture or if more diffuse periostitis. Chronic periostitis is often associated with palpable firm bumpy uneven texture along the midportion of the tibia. The posterior medial border of the tibia is palpable by digging the fingers around behind the medial border, carefully probing the posterior aspect of the tibia can help to identify stress fractures of the posterior cortex which can present as calf pain with or without shin pain. After palpating the distal aspect of the posterior tibia, examination should extend into the foot to probe the navicular tubercle. The navicular tubercle is the insertion of the posterior tibialis, and pathology of the navicular can often give rise to medial ankle and leg pain.

Bony palpation of the posterior leg is limited to the flabella of the lateral gastrocnemius tendon and posterior ankle. In the ankle, the posterior talus and dome of the calcaneus should be examined. The dome of the calcaneus and posterior talus are palpated in the soft depression just anterior to the Achilles tendon. Pain with bony palpation of the calcaneus can suggest fracture, stress injury, or in adolescents—calcaneal apophysitis. Compression of the calcaneus for each side, the so-called squeeze test, can help evaluate for bony pain. The pain with palpation of the posterior talus suggests possible posterior malleolus fracture, os trigonum syndrome, or posterior impingement syndrome. Deformities of the calcaneus and soft tissue calcification should be noted and palpated for tenderness. A Haglund's deformity presents as a distinct bony prominence of the posterolateral calcaneus. This should be distinguished from Haglund's disease which results from soft tissue inflammation of the retrocalcaneal bursa and Achilles tendon insertion. Enthesophytes or spurring at the insertion of the calcaneus is common and may be associated with pain on palpation.

Bony palpation of the lateral aspect of the leg should begin at the lateral joint line extending along the lateral tibial plateau to head of the fibula. Instability, arthritis, or ganglions of superior tibiofibular joint often present as pain in the lateral calf or leg. Continuing distally an attempt should be made to palpate the entire length of the fibula to the lateral malleolus. Focal pain with palpation of the fibula without a history of trauma suggests stress fracture, injuries that often refer pain to the posterior or lateral leg. The proximal fibula can also be fractured from a direct blow or following significant rotation ankle sprains that result in propagation of a Maisonneuve fracture.

Soft Tissue Palpation

Soft tissue palpation is often the most valuable part of the clinical examination for posterior leg pain. When you are familiar with the natural history of muscle injuries in the posterior leg, hear the patients' account of their pain and observe them walk into the exam room; anatomical-based palpation can often quickly allow the examiner to literal and figuratively *put their finger on the problem*. Although this is very rewarding, it is critical to complete the exam to evaluate for any concomitant pathology and assess for causative factors.

It is important to palpate the soft tissue structures in their entirety. In respect to muscles, the whole muscle belly as well as the associated tendons and aponeurosis should be carefully examined for trigger points, increased tone, swelling, thickening, defect, or mass. It is helpful to palpate in both a relaxed state and during active contraction. Palpating though the full range of relative joint motion can aid evaluation of symptomatic muscles. In addition, some soft tissue palpation is best done after exertion. This is particularly helpful to evaluate for muscle herniations and chronic compartment syndrome where the palpation of the can be normal at rest but become tight, tender, and swollen with extended exertion.

To perform a comprehensive examination of the leg by palpation, it is helpful to proceed in a sequential fashion. Begin with the posterior aspect of the knee. Here the popliteal fossa can be a good landmark to help define the relevant structures. The superior borders of the popliteal fossa are bound by the biceps femoris tendon laterally and the semimembranous and semitendinosus muscle medially. From this location, distal biceps femoris should be palpated to its attachment on the posterior fibula and the medial hamstring tendons along the posterior medial knee to their respective attachments. The semitendinosus tendon travels medially with the sartorius and gracilis to form the combined pes anserine insertion. The location of the pes anserine is a common site of bursitis on the anterior medial leg but which can extend posteriorly causing leg pain and swelling.

The inferior margins of the fossa are formed by the medial and lateral heads of the gastrocnemius. When present, the plantaris muscle belly will be palpable medial to the lateral head of the gastrocnemius in the popliteal fossa. A neurovascular bundle containing the popliteal artery, vein, and posterior tibial nerve cross through the popliteal area from deep to superficial, respectively.

With the knee in a relaxed and flexed position, the popliteal artery pulse can usually be felt by pressing the fingers deep into the fossa along the posterior joint capsule of the knee. Absence or asymmetrical palpation of the popliteal pulse can suggest vascular occlusive disease or mechanical obstruction. Because it is the most superficial structure crossing the popliteal area, occasionally disorders of the posterior tibial nerve can result in a palpable neuroma or positive compression test for neuritis. The tibial nerve provides muscle and sensory innervation to the posterior leg. Isolated tibial neuropathy is uncommon but can arise from a schwannoma or direct compression from a popliteal mass such as a baker's cyst, popliteal aneurysm, or hematoma.

The saphenous nerve supplies sensation to the medial leg. Saphenous nerve injury can be an isolated finding or related to femoral neuropathy. An isolated injury to the saphenous nerve will produce only sensory deficits. The saphenous nerve can be injured during knee surgery, venous grafting for coronary artery bypass, or from direct trauma. Injuries to the saphenous nerve can lead to tenderness or paresthesias in the medial leg. The infrapatella branch of the saphenous nerve can be palpated over the medial tibia at the level of the tibial tubercle. A positive Tinel's sign can help confirm the diagnosis by briskly tapping along the nerve to reproduce symptoms.

Popliteal (Baker's) cysts are a common finding on palpation of the popliteal fossa. Classically, Baker's cysts will occur at the medial aspect of the fossa between the medial gastrocnemius and semimembranosus tendons and are more easily palpable with the knee in extension. Often Baker's cysts will be asymptomatic and represent an incidental finding. However, when Baker's cysts are symptomatic they can cause posterior leg pain or sensations of swelling and tightness in the calf that are exacerbated by activity or prolonged standing. Baker's cysts are prone to leakage or rupture which can produce acute, severe pain and swelling in the posterior leg. A ruptured Baker's cyst is often misdiagnosed as a DVT or gastrocnemius strain.

Although they can have loculated segments, Baker's cysts arise from invaginations of the knee joint synovia and communicate with the knee joint. Occasionally, Baker's cysts will become vastly distended and cause a palpable mass in the calf. Conditions that produce effusions of the knee will result in progressive enlargement of the cyst. Therefore, treatment of symptomatic Baker's cysts is best accomplished by treating the underlying pathology of the knee that results in increased synovial fluid production. In certain circumstances, drainage or surgical resection of the cyst can be considered.

Moving distal from the popliteal fossa the most superficial structure of the posterior leg is the gastrocnemius. The gastrocnemius extends from above the knee to its insertion on the calcaneus. The muscle can be palpated in a relaxed position when the knee is in flexion. Increased muscle tone and thickened bands of tissue suggest abnormal tightness and may predispose to strain. Findings of contracture or excessive tightness should prompt investigation of causative factors such as poor biomechanics. Chronic strains often result in fibrotic disorganized scar tissue that can frequently be detected on careful palpation. Contusions of the gastrocnemius can reveal palpable hematoma and swelling. Acute strains of the gastrocnemius most commonly occur at the belly or distal myotendinous junction of the medial head of the gastrocnemius and are often associated with significant swelling and ecchymosis. Increased tone, marked tenderness, and a palpable hematoma can often be easily appreciated. In high-grade tears, a palpable defect in the muscle is present. Stretching or contraction of the gastrocnemius during palpation aggravates symptoms.

The soleus lies deep to the gastrocnemius. A pincer grip allows for palpation of the medial and lateral borders of the soleus deep to the gastrocnemius. The medial third of the soleus can become noticeably hard and inflexible often in association with increased subtalar pronation. The soleus aponeurosis can be easily palpated in the distal posterior leg. Tender ropy texture of the aponeurosis is often associated with medial shin pain. Strains of the soleus are typically found in the lateral portion of the muscle. Palpation of the lateral soleus deep to the gastrocnemius will reveal tenderness and increased tone which wors-

ens with passive stretch and active contraction of the muscle.

An accessory soleus is an anatomical variant estimated to be present in 5 % of the population [4]. Most commonly it presents as a palpable unilateral soft tissue mass or visible asymmetrical fullness in distal medial aspect of the posterior leg. An accessory soleus muscle can be painful and lead to posterior tibial nerve compression or compartment syndrome.

The gastrocnemius, soleus, and plantaris share a common attachment on the calcaneus by way of the Achilles tendon. The Achilles tendon is a thick, superficial, and easily palpable from the distal one third of the calf to the calcaneus. The tendon is a common source of posterior leg pain and should be carefully examined along its length for thickening, crepitus, calcific densities, defects, and pain. The most common cause of Achilles tendon pain is due to tendinopathy, but it is also frequently strained or ruptured.

Achilles tendinopathy can be insidious in onset but is typically associated with abrupt changes in activity. Achilles tendinopathy can be found in both the midportion of the tendon or at its insertion. Midsubstance Achilles tendinopathy is characterized by tenderness on palpation of the midportion of the tendon often associated with nodular thickening, swelling, or crepitus. Calcific deposits within the midportion of the tendon can occur and, if present, are typical easily palpable and visible on x-ray. Insertional Achilles tendinopathy is found along the broad insertion of the Achilles at the calcaneus. Insertional Achilles tendinopathy is often associated with a Haglund's deformity, retrocalcaneal or calcaneal bursitis, and enthesophyte formation.

Achilles tendon rupture is a common injury in male middle-aged athletes. Patients often report thinking they were struck in the back of the leg and heard a snap or pop associated with acute loss of the push-off phase of gait. Acutely, a visible and palpable defect is typically present about 2 in. proximal to the Achilles tendon insertion. However, with time the defect may be masked by swelling. Examination is best performed with the patient prone and feet off the examination table. A combination of findings on inspection, palpation, and manual muscle testing along with a positive Thomson test is used to make the diagnosis. The Thomson test is typically performed with the patient prone on the exam table so that the knee is fully extended and the ankle off the table in a relaxed neutral position. The midportion of the calf is then squeezed to produce plantar flexion. A positive test will result in markedly decreased or absent motion.

The deep posterior compartment of the leg contains the tibialis posterior, flexor digitorum longus, and flexor hallucis longus muscles as well as two separate vascular bundles comprising the tibial nerve and posterior tibial vessels as well as fibular artery and vein, respectively. Effective palpation of the deep posterior compartment of the leg requires the muscle of the superficial posterior compartment to be relaxed. This can be accomplished by passive flexion of the knee and plantar flexion of the ankle with the patient in a seated or prone position. Using a hook-type grip, the posterior compartment can then be examined from the posterior medial aspect of the tibia deep to the soleus. Tightness, pain, or palpable masses due to muscle herniations should be sought. Examination of the deep posterior compartment should extend to palpation of the tendons of the deep compartment as the pass behind the medial malleus and to their insertions (see Fig. 10.1 in Chap. 10). The popliteus muscle has its origin as a tendinous attachment on the lateral femoral condyle and posterior lateral horn of the meniscus. It inserts more broadly along posterior tibial above the soleus and deep to the gastrocnemius and plantaris. The popliteus assists in knee flexion and internal rotation of the leg. It can be palpated at both its origin and insertion. This is best accomplished in the prone position with the knee flexed. By palpating or pining the muscle while alternating between a shortened position (passive knee flexion and internal rotation of the leg) and lengthened position (passive knee extension and external rotation of the leg) pain arising from the popliteus can be more accurately reproduced. Injuries of the popliteus can be isolated but more often are associated with posterior lateral corner injures in the knee. Symptoms of popliteus injury

included limited ROM, knee instability, and posterior leg pain [5].

Along the fibular head and neck, the common peroneal nerve is vulnerable to injury and compression. Neuropathy of the common peroneal nerve can result weakness in ankle dorsiflexion and eversion with pain and paresthesias in the posterior lateral leg and dorsum of the foot. Manual compression or a Tinel's test of the nerve at this location should reproduce or aggravate symptoms.

Range of Motion Testing for Posterior Leg Pain

There is variation on the reported normal ROM values for adults [6–8]. For example, reported normal knee flexion ranges from 130 to 160°, while ankle dorsiflexion normal values have been reported from 13 to 30°. In the clinical setting ROM is often estimated, but use of a universal goniometer can be helpful in establishing the experience to make accurate estimates or in case where specific measurement is helpful. Universal goniometers are common in orthopedic or rehab clinics. They consist of a protractor augmented by two ruler-like arms, one arm is fixed or stationary while the other arm is mobile or moving. The fulcrum of the goniometer is placed at the axis of motion of the joint that you want to measure. The fixed arm is aligned in parallel with the long axis of the limb segment that is proximal to the joint ROM being measured. The moving arm is attached by a rivet rotates around the center of the protractor and is aligned with the limb segment that is distal to the joint ROM being measured. Given the range of normal values it is helpful to make side to side comparison in determining deviations from normal for a given patient.

Normal ROM values for the distal lower extremity are as follows: Knee flexion ranges from 130 to 160°. Ankle dorsiflexion normal values have been reported from 13 to 30° while ankle plantar flexion has reported normal values from 45 to 56°. The subtalar joint ROM has a wide range of normal values reported for inversion 5–52° and eversion 5–30° of motion. The transverse tarsal motion range of normal values includes 20–50° of inversion and 10–20° of eversion. First toe metatarsophalangeal (MTP) motion is reported at 30–45° flexion and 40–90° extension. While the lesser toes MTP ROM is 35–40° of flexion and 40° of extension.

It is important to consider both active and passive ROM. If active ROM is limited, passive ROM testing can provide significant clinical information. When active ROM is significantly less than passive ROM, it indicates limitations are likely from patient guarding, soft tissue pathology such as muscle injury or tendon rupture. In passive ROM "end feel" is often reported and can be a helpful aid to the clinician. End feel is usually described as hard or soft. Hard end feel typically is used to describe bony obstruction to further ROM. Hard end feel in the setting of abnormal passive ROM often indicates bony impingement or other static restriction to motion such as joint contractures. Soft end feel is more of a stiffness of the tissues and can be due to increased neural tone, guarding, or passive properties of the soft tissues themselves.

Manual Muscle Testing of the Posterior Leg

Manual muscle testing is a critical part of the examination of the posterior leg. Because the muscles of the posterior leg are all predominately plantar flexors, weakness of the muscles of the posterior leg can result in similar functional complaints. Therefore, isolation of individual muscle function on manual muscle testing is particularly important for determining the underlying pathology. Weakness on manual muscle testing can result from structural, neuropathic, or patient-mediated causes. It is important to know both the neurologic innervation and function of each of the muscle in the posterior leg. In addition, if pain or guarding significantly limits the exam, detailed conclusions from manual muscle testing will be tenuous.

The gastrocnemius, soleus, and plantaris make up the superficial posterior compartment

of the leg. They share a common innervation (S1, S2, and tibial nerve) and tendon (Achilles) insertion on the calcaneus and all contribute to plantar flexion of the ankle. Of these muscles, the gastrocnemius has a disproportional influence on ankle plantarflexion and therefore can make it challenging to assess the contribution of the soleus and plantaris on manual muscle testing. In addition, because of the large size of the gastrocnemius subtle weakness will be difficult to identify on standard manual muscle testing. To address these issues, the isolation of the gastrocnemius can be improved during manual muscle testing by having the patient plantar flex the ankle against resistance with the knee in extension and the ankle in dorsiflexion. This can initially be done with the patient seated. If strength is full and pain free, the patient can be placed supine on the examination table with the knee fully extending while you position yourself to use your body weight to provide additional resistance plantar flexion. Single leg heel raises with the knee extended can also reveal subtle weakness in the gastrocnemius.

Like the gastrocnemius, the plantaris cross both the knee and ankle. The plantaris plays a minimal role in ankle plantar flexion. For these reasons, isolation of the plantaris from the gastrocnemius on manual muscle testing is largely untenable. For a suspected plantaris rupture, manual muscle testing for the plantaris should be done, such as the gastrocnemius, with the knee in an extended position. The muscle belly of the plantaris is located adjacent to the lateral head of the gastrocnemius in the popliteal fossa. Most gastrocnemius injuries occur in the medial head, so if manual muscle produces pain or cramping in the posterior lateral leg at the level of the popliteal fossa it may suggest plantaris injury.

Unlike the gastrocnemius and plantaris, the soleus does not cross the knee joint. Therefore, manual muscle testing of the soleus should be performed with the knee in flexion and the ankle in dorsiflexion to limit the contribution of the gastrocnemius in plantar flexion. Most soleus strains occur laterally at the myotendinous junction.

The deep posterior compartment of the leg contains the posterior tibialis, flexor hallucis longus, and flexor digitorum. All three muscles are predominantly innervated by L5 and the tibial nerve. The posterior tibialis is a plantar flexor and supinator of the ankle. The posterior tibialis can be difficult to isolate in manual muscle testing. Testing can be facilitated by placing the ankle in eversion and having the patient plantar flex and invert the ankle against resistance. A modified heel raise can also be used to test the strength of the posterior tibialis. Have the patient stand as close as possible to the wall and then perform a single leg heel rise with their weight centered over the medial aspect of the foot and great toe. The flexor hallucis longus muscle can be manually tested by having the patient plantar flex or curl the great toe against resistance while you stabilize the calcaneus. Likewise, the flexor digitorum longus muscle can be tested stabilizing the heel and having the patient plantar flex or curl the lesser toes.

The Neurologic Examination for Posterior Leg Pain

Neuromyofascial pathology can cause referred pain to the posterior leg. As noted in the section on manual muscle testing, weakness can be caused from orthopedic or neurologic abnormalities. Sensation and manual muscle testing should be performed in all patients to evaluate for neuropathy. In addition, trigger points in the gluteal muscles have been described as frequent cause of referred pain to the posterior leg. The joints of the spine and associated soft tissue have also been implicated as a potential cause of referred pain to the posterior leg. Patients with intermittent posterior leg pain that is variable in location and character should prompt the clinician to consider referred pain from neuromyofascial causes. Chapter 13, *Complementary Medicine Practices for Muscular Injuries of the Posterior Lower Leg* contains a detailed discussion of the evaluation and management of posterior leg pain from myofascial causes.

As discussed above, peripheral nerve entrapments can cause posterior leg pain. Sural nerve entrapment can result from trauma such as surgery or compression from a cast. Sural nerve entrapment can also be caused internal compression due to mass or swelling. Tibial nerve entrapment is an infrequent cause of leg pain. However, tibial nerve entrapment can occur due to compression from a Baker's cyst, popliteal artery aneurysm, or other space occupying mass. Tibial neuropathy can lead to paresthesias of the plantar surface of the foot and weakness in ankle plantar flexion, inversion, and toe flexion.

Patients with chronic or intermittent posterior leg pain, particularly if associated with myotomal weakness and dermatomal paresthesias should be carefully examined for lumbar radicular pathology. Radiculopathy from L4, L5, S1, and S2 nerve roots can all refer pain to the posterior leg. Characteristically L4 radiculopathy is associated medial leg pain, while L5 radiculopathy can cause lateral leg pain and S1 or S2 more classic calf pain. Patients with radiculopathy will typically have correlated myotomal weakness and sensory disturbances. Pathology at the L4 neurologic level is associated with weakness in ankle dorsiflexion, abnormalities in patellar reflex testing, and sensory abnormalities along the medial ankle and foot. L5 radiculopathy is associated with weakness in the extensor hallucis longus and posterior tibialis. Sensory loss associated with L5 radiculopahty is seen in the lateral leg, dorsum of the foot and web space between the 1st and 2nd toes. There is no associated reflex testing for L5 radiculopathy. Lumbar radiculopathy from the S1 nerve root is associated with weakness in ankle eversion and plantar flexion making toe walking symptomatic. Sensory abnormities occur over the lateral foot and heel. Abnormal Achilles reflexes are also associated with S1 radiculopathy. Of note, S2 radiculopathy cannot be directly assessed from the lower extremity examination but can affect the intrinsic muscles of the foot resulting in dysfunction of deformity.

Several neural dynamic tests have been described to help the clinician assess for neurogenic pain. These tests attempt to isolate and stress the neural structures to reproduce or aggravate the patients presenting complaints. The straight leg test is used to induce back and leg pain in patients with suspected radiculopathy. To perform the straight leg test, have the patient lie supine on the examination table with the knees fully extended and neck in neutral position. The examiner should cup the heel of the affected extremity and then passively lift it off the table while maintaining full knee extension. The extremity should be raised until symptoms are produced or passive ROM is constrained. A positive test reproduces or aggravates the patient's leg pain or neurologic symptoms. The positive straight leg test is often associated with discomfort in the lumbar spine or along the course of the sciatic nerve. The Kerning test is used to increase tension on the spinal cord and associated soft tissue. The Kerning test is performed by having the patient actively move chin to chest from a supine position with both hands placed behind the head. The patient should maintain a maximally forward flexed position; if no pain in the neck is experienced by the patient with active flexion, the examiner can apply gentle overpressure to increase the stretch. A positive test reproduces back and leg pain.

The slump test is a neural dynamic test that combines elements of the straight leg raise and Kerning test to increase the tension on neural tissue. The slump test can be very effective in revealing if the patient's leg pain has a neural component. Many variations of the slump test are possible, but the general principle is to progressively increase the neural tissue tension to a point of maximal stretch by means of spinal flexion, extension of the knee, and dorsiflexion of the ankle. The slump test is typically performed with the patient seated on the exam table with the thigh supported and the knee in relaxed flexion. To begin the test, the patient slumps forward at the waist and shoulders, then the patient actively forward flexes the neck so that the chin rests on the chest at which point the patient actively extends one knee and finally actively dorsiflexes the ipsilateral ankle. During this sequence of movements the examiner assesses for replication or aggravation of the patients presenting complaint and the onset of other symptoms that would suggest neuropathic pain. If symptoms are produced with neural tension, then the examiner should assess if they are likewise relieved

by reducing neural tension and the degree to which each component movement produces or relieves symptoms. A positive test reproduces the patient's symptoms and responds consistently to increased or decreased neural tension [9].

Calf cramps are a common and painful occurrence. Although a variety of etiologies for muscle cramps have been proposed [10]. However, a general consensus is building that calf cramps arise due to alterations in spinal neural reflex activity. This deregulation seems to be mediated by fatigue and environmental factors in susceptible individuals. Calf cramps can occur at rest and are frequently nocturnal. Calf cramps are also regularly seen in athletes during intense activity and are often associated with fluid balance or environmental factors.

The Vascular Examination for Posterior Leg Pain

Vascular disorders can cause posterior leg pain. Most posterior leg pain from vascular origin presents as claudication or positional pain. However, occasionally painful masses found in the posterior leg can be from vascular causes [11, 12]. Incidental findings of vascular calcification on routine x-ray imaging should prompt greater concern for potential vascular pathology. There is significant overlap between posterior leg pain caused by vascular etiologies, exertional compartment syndromes, and neurogenic causes. Clinical evaluation of the vascular system can be helpful in discriminating between these diagnoses. However, evaluation can be challenging during routine examination as findings are often present only after provocation by specific activities. For this reason, clinical testing should be done both at rest and dynamic states if a vascular disorder is suspected. Despite the importance of the clinical exam, imaging studies or other testing is often required to confirm the vascular causes of leg pain. More information on imaging and tests for vascular disorders can be found in Chap. 7, *Imaging and Tests for Assessment of the Posterior Leg.*

Vascular Entrapments

Vascular entrapments are an uncommon cause of posterior leg pain and can be difficult to diagnosis. However, they remain an important consideration in patients presenting with activity-induced posterior leg pain. Vascular entrapment presents as exertional leg pain that resolves promptly with rest. A repetitive exercise bout on consecutive days does not result in more severe symptoms. Pain can be worse with walking than running. Occasionally vascular entrapment is associated with signs of acute or chronic limb ischemia. Popliteal artery entrapment can be anatomical or functional. Anatomical entrapment occurs due to structural variation in the course of the popliteal artery or constriction from the presence of abnormal soft tissue structures. Functional popliteal artery entrapment is thought to be related to hypertrophy of the gastrocnemius that result in compression of the artery during active plantar flexion of the ankle. Entrapment of the anterior tibial artery has been reported at the interosseous membrane of the tibia and fibula.

The clinical examination for vascular entrapments often requires reproducing the action that causes the entrapment. Examination of pulses immediate postexercise can reveal weak or absent distal pulses. Palpation of pulses during passive dorsiflexion and active plantar flexion of the ankle can produce dynamic deficits in popliteal pulse suggesting possible entrapment. Likewise, auscultation of a bruit is occasionally found at rest but is more likely to be elicited in dynamic position with maximal active contraction of the gastrocnemius or passive dorsiflexion of the ankle. Similarly, an ankle brachial index (ABI) in dynamic position can be used to evaluate for dynamic vascular entrapment.

Chronic Exertional Compartment

Chronic exertional compartment syndrome is characterized by complaints of bilateral leg pain that develops at particular intensity or duration of exercise and resolves gradually within 30 min of ceasing activity. Often symptoms worsen with repeat bouts of the offending activity on consecutive days and can progress to the point of developing weakness, paresthesias, or rest pain in severe cases. Although chronic exertional compartment syndrome is most commonly found in the anterior and lateral compartments of the leg, deep compartment syndrome is an important cause of chronic exertional posterior leg pain. Compartment syndrome of the superficial posterior compartment of the leg is rare but can be a cause of posterior leg pain. On examination, the affected compartments can look and feel tight. When symptoms of chronic exertional compartment syndrome are precipitated through exercise the effected compartments are noticeably taut and tender to palpation. Examination after exercise often reveals weakness of the involved muscles and occasionally paresthesias on the plantar aspect of foot from tibial nerve compression. Palpation of posterior tibial pulse both pre- and postexercise should be performed to evaluate for dynamic change. Definitive diagnosis of chronic exertional compartment syndrome is made by direct testing of the intracompartmental pressure. Testing and treatment of chronic exertional compartment syndrome is discussed in Chaps. 7 and 10, respectively.

Vascular Claudication

Atherosclerotic vessel disease or end-artery stenosis can lead to posterior leg pain. Although most common in sedentary older patients with a history of peripheral vascular disease, atherosclerosis or end-artery stenosis can mimic gastrocnemius strain or present as subtle exertional leg pain in athletes [13]. Vascular claudication should be considered in masters athletes who present with caudation, particularly if vascular calcification is noted on x-rays or if examination reveals stigmata of vascular disease. Stigmata of vascular disease are suggested by thickened nails, reduced or absent hair, shiny skin. The palpation of pulses is often reduced or absent. Auscultation of an arterial bruit at rest or postexercise suggests turbulent flow from vascular obstruction. In patients with suspected peripheral vascular disease, an ABI should be obtained at rest and if necessary postexercise. Vascular disease that results in abnormal stiffening of the vessel can produce a false negative or an abnormally elevated ABI— so-called noncompressible disease. If extensive vascular calcification is noted on x-ray or abnormally elevated values are obtained by ABI, further investigations should be considered.

Endofibrosis

Arterial endofibrosis can cause exertional posterior leg pain but most commonly presents in the thigh. The pathology appears to have a proclivity for endurance athletes who engage in repetitive hip flexion which leads to repetitive kinking and microtrauma of the artery. Most common in cyclists, arterial endofibrosis has also been reported in runners, rowers, rugby players, race walkers, and triathletes. Symptoms typically present as unilateral cramping or tightness of the lower extremity during intense exercise progressing rapidly to cause reduction or cessation of activity. The vast majority of arterial endofibrosis is found in iliac artery but has also been described in proximal and distal distributions. Psoas hypertrophy and heredity factors have been suggested as possible predisposing causes to development of endofibrosis. Clinical examination for arterial endofibrosis includes auscultation for bruits over femoral artery during dynamic positioning of the hip in flexion at rest or immediately postexercise and palpation of distal weak or absent pulses immediately after exercise. ABI testing done at rest and postexercise can be used to augment the clinical evaluation. Definitive diagnosis is made by vascular imaging.

Deep Venous Thrombosis

DVT can present as posterior leg pain or can arise as a complication of injuries to the leg. Risk factors include trauma, immobilization, and clotting disorders. The trauma, reduced use, and swelling that result in muscle injuries to the posterior leg, all increase the risk of DVT and should inform thoughtful recommendations for the treatment of the primary injury to reduce the chance of this complication. DVT is a relatively common complication of lower extremity surgery, and patients presenting with posterior leg pain after surgery should engender a high index of suspicion for this disorder [14]. DVT typically presents as posterior leg pain and swelling associated with increased warmth and calf tenderness. Homan's sign is a clinical examination test that is often performed to assess for DVT. A positive Homan's sign elicits pain in the calf during forceful overpressure of passive dorsiflexion of the ankle with the knee in full extension. Diagnosis of DVT can be made with the assistance of laboratory and imaging tests.

Additional Special Tests for Posterior Leg Pain

Assessment of Leg Length Discrepancy

If inspection suggests possible leg length discrepancy, further clinical evaluation can be performed to identify the asymmetry. With the patient lying supine in neutral position and with the legs fully supported by the table, compare the relative position of the medial malleoli of each ankle. If a significant difference is noted between the two legs, further tests for leg length asymmetries can help determine if the leg length discrepancy is anatomical or functional.

Anatomical discrepancies can be found by measuring the length of each leg and evaluating the individual segments. Measurement of leg length is typically performed supine, with the legs symmetrically positioned and fully supported on the table. From this position, a tape measure is used to determine the distance from the anterior superior iliac spine (ASIS) to the medial malleolus of each leg. If a substantial difference is identified between the two legs, the segmental lengths of the femur and tibia can be assessed quickly by moving the patient's legs so that the knees are flexed to 90° with the feet together, heels parallel and flat on the table. Tibial length differences can then be evaluated by looking up from the foot of the bed and checking to see if one knee extends higher than the other. Asymmetry of femur length is assessed by viewing the knees from the side to see if one knee juts ahead of the other.

Functional or apparent leg length discrepancies arise from asymmetries at the hip or pelvis. Measurements for anatomical leg length as described above should be independent of any functional or apparent leg length discrepancy. If functional leg length is suspected, a measurement from umbilicus to each medial malleoli can determine the amount of the leg length discrepancy. Functional leg length asymmetry often results from pelvic obliquity; if this is the case a trial of manual techniques to correct the pelvic obliquity can often improve or resolve the discrepancy.

Silfverskiold Test

The Silfverskiold test is used to determine if an equinus contracture arises from the gastrocnemius or the Achilles tendon. The test is performed by holding the hindfoot in neutral position while testing the range of ankle dorsiflexion with the knee in full extension and subsequently at 90° of flexion. If additional dorsiflexion is noted with the knee in flexion then the contracture involves the gastrocnemius (see Fig. 10.2 in Chap. 10).

Tuning Fork Test for Stress Fractures

A tuning fork can be used to percuss along the tibia and portions of the fibula as a clinical assessment for stress fracture. Although the evidence for the tuning fork test is questionable, it is easily applied in a clinical setting and if positive may expedite treatment while definitive diagnosis is pending [15, 16]. Typically this test is done after identifying areas of bony tenderness on palpation. To perform the test, the tuning fork is struck and then placed on the previously identified site of bony tenderness. If the vibrations from the tuning fork elicit pain this would be considered a positive test.

References

1. Physician Visits: Reason for Visit—Based on data from the National Ambulatory Medical Care Survey, 2000–2010; National Center for Health Statistics. Rosemont: Department of Research & Scientific Affairs, American Academy of Orthopaedic Surgeons (AAOS); 2013.
2. Neal BS, Griffiths IB, Dowling GJ, Murley GS, Munteanu SE, Franettovich Smith MM, Collins NJ, Barton CJ. Foot posture as a risk factor for lower limb overuse injury: a systematic review and meta-analysis. J Foot Ankle Res. 2014;7(1):55.
3. Dowling GJ, Murley GS, Munteanu SE, Smith MM, Neal BS, Griffiths IB, Barton CJ, Collins NJ. Dynamic foot function as a risk factor for lower limb overuse injury: a systematic review. J Foot Ankle Res. 2014;7(1):53.
4. Christodoulou A, Terzidis I, Natsis K, et al. Soleus accessories, an anomalous muscle in a young athlete: case report and analysis of the literature. Br J Sports Med. 2004;38:e38.
5. Nyland J, Lachman N, Kocabey Y, Brosky J, Altun R, Caborn D. Anatomy, function, and rehabilitation of the popliteus musculotendinous complex. J Orthop Sports Phys Ther. 2005;35(3):165–79.
6. Boone DC, Azen SP. Normal range of motion of joints in male subjects. J Bone Joint Surg Am. 1979;61(5):756–9.
7. Roaas A, Andersson GB. Normal range of motion of the hip, knee and ankle joints in male subjects, 30–40 years of age. Acta Orthop. 1982;53(2):205–8.
8. Gajdosik RL, Bohannon RW. Clinical measurement of range of motion. Review of goniometry emphasizing reliability and validity. Phys Ther. 1987;67(12):1867–72.
9. Majlesi J, Togay H, Unalan H, Toprak S. The sensitivity and specificity of the slump and the straight leg raising tests in patients with lumbar disc herniation. J Clin Rheumatol. 2008;14(2):87–91.
10. Minetto MA, Holobar A, Botter A, Farina D. Origin and development of muscle cramps. Exerc Sport Sci Rev. 2013;41(1):3–10.
11. Hristov N, Atanasov Z, Zafirovski G, Mitrev Z. Intramuscular cavernous hemangioma in the left soleus muscle: successful surgical treatment. Interact Cardiovasc Thorac Surg. 2011;13(5):521–2.
12. Wierzbicki JM, Henderson JH, Scarborough MT, Bush CH, Reith JD, Clugston JR. Intramuscular hemangiomas. Sports Health. 2013;5(5):448–54.
13. Lundgren JM, Davis BA. Endartery stenosis of the popliteal artery mimicking gastrocnemius strain: a case report. Arch Phys Med Rehabil. 2004;85:1548–51.
14. Sun Y, Chen D, Xu Z, Shi D, Dai J, Qin J, Qin J, Jiang Q. Deep venous thrombosis after knee arthroscopy: a systematic review and meta-analysis. Arthroscopy. 2014;30(3):406–12.

15. Schneiders AG, Sullivan SJ, Hendrick PA, Hones BD, McMaster AR, Sugden BA, Tomlinson C. The ability of clinical tests to diagnose stress fractures: a systematic review and meta-analysis. J Orthop Sports Phys Ther. 2012;42(9):760–71.
16. Fatima ST, Jeilani A, Mazhar-ud-Duha, Abbasi NZ, Khan AA, Khan K, Sheikh AS, Ali F, Memon KH. Validation of tuning fork test in stress fractures and its comparison with radionuclide bone scan. J Ayub Med Coll Abbottabad. 2012;24(3–4):180–2.
17. Shinohara N, Nagano S, Yokouchi M, Arishima Y, Tabata K, Higashi M, Kitajima S, Yonezawa S, Komiya S. Bilobular calcifying fibrous pseudotumor in soleus muscle: a case report. J Med Case Rep. 2011;5:487.

Imaging and Tests for Posterior Lower Leg

Eric P. Sturos and J. Bryan Dixon

Introduction

Posterior leg pain has a wide variety of causes, many of which can be difficult to determine clinically. Several diagnostic tests are available to assist the clinician in confirming the diagnosis of a muscle injury and evaluating for other etiologies of posterior leg pain. The main focus of this chapter will be on magnetic resonance imaging (MRI) and ultrasonography, as these tests are widely available and particularly helpful in diagnosing soft tissue injuries. This chapter is organized into sections covering musculoskeletal injuries, impairments of the nervous system, vascular disorders, and a more wide-ranging section regarding tests for other etiologies of posterior leg pain.

Musculoskeletal Injuries

MRI and ultrasound (US) are currently considered the modality of choice in the imaging of musculotendinous injuries [1]. Radiographs are frequently the first imaging modality used in the assessment of leg pain and are particularly helpful in evaluating skeletal abnormalities, but play a limited role in suspected soft tissue injuries [2]. Because of the limited role diagnostic X-ray and computed tomography (CT) play in evaluating soft tissue injuries, these modalities will not be covered in detail but the reader should keep in mind the usefulness of these tests in evaluating patients for fractures, heterotopic ossification, tumors, and other bony abnormalities that are in the differential diagnosis of posterior leg pain.

Athletes and active people are at high risk for muscle injury of the posterior leg due to the demands of their sport or occupational activities [1]. Muscle injuries are common in athletes with over 90 % of the muscle injuries caused by excessive strain or contusion [3]. Although injuries to the posterior leg can often be diagnosed clinically, imaging has an important role in determining management, optimizing rehabilitation, and differentiating musculotendinous injury from other causes of posterior leg pain. Imaging studies are also commonly used if a definitive diagnosis cannot be made with the history and physical exam or if prognostic information is needed to guide *return to play expectations* for elite athletes.

Common injuries to the musculotendinous units in the posterior leg include strain, contusion, and avulsion injuries. These injuries are generally characterized by muscle fiber disruption, intramuscular hemorrhagic dissection, hematoma around the fascia or at the muscle-tendon

E. P. Sturos (✉)
Department of Physical Medicine and Rehabilitation, Vanderbilt University School of Medicine, Nashville, TN, USA
e-mail: ericsturos@gmail.com

J. B. Dixon
Sports Medicine, Advanced Center for Orthopedics, Marquette, MI, USA
e-mail: jbryandixon@hotmail.com

junction, and in the case of avulsion, separation of a tendon or ligament from its bony attachment. Each of these injuries is described below to assist the reader in determining which studies to order, how to interpret the results and to elucidate the role of imaging in follow-up to the acute injury.

Muscle Strain, Tear, and Rupture

Muscle strains or tears often affect muscles that have primarily fast-twitch type-2 muscle fibers, span two joints, and undergo eccentric contraction [3]. The gastrocnemius muscle has all of these risk factors for injury and, not surprisingly, is the most frequently injured muscle in the posterior leg. The soleus is considered low risk because it only crosses the ankle joint and is largely made up of slow-twitch type-1 fibers. When a muscle is subjected to stresses beyond its capacity, injury will occur at the weakest point along the muscle–tendon–bone axis. In adults, the myotendinous junction is commonly the weakest point on this axis and is therefore the location of most strains, tears, and ruptures.

In the case of a suspected muscle strain, diagnostic imaging can be used to confirm the diagnosis, provide detailed information on the degree of injury, aid in surgical planning, evaluate for alternative or concomitant pathology, and provide information to guide conservative treatment and return to play expectations. Ultrasound and MRI are particularly well suited to the evaluation of myotendinous injury. The choice between these imaging modalities varies based on a variety of factors [3].

If used by an experienced operator, ultrasound is an ideal choice for imaging acute muscle injuries of the posterior leg [4]. In acute injuries, the clinical exam is often limited by pain and swelling. Ultrasound can often be used in this situation to make a rapid and accurate diagnosis. Ultrasound also has the advantages of portability, ease of use, and decreased cost when compared to MRI. Ultrasound has excellent dynamic spatial resolution but it can be difficult to visual the deep structures of the leg, is less widely available, and more operator dependent than MRI.

Ultrasound is generally thought to be inferior to MRI in the sub-acute and chronic phases when the injury-related edema starts to resolve [3]. MRI is more expensive but has superior soft tissue contrast, excellent spatial resolution, and reproducibility.

Ultrasound

Musculoskeletal diagnostic ultrasonography is inexpensive and available in most settings that offer specialty radiological or sports medicine services. It allows for dynamic imaging which can provide unique and valuable information to aid in diagnosis [1]. In addition, ultrasound's ability to provide real-time visualization makes it ideal for guiding interventional procedures such as aspirations or injections. Ultrasound, however, remains operator dependent and is generally considered inferior to MRI in follow-up imaging due to its inability to differentiate the acuity of lesions, and the difficulty in reproducing the exact same position/plane of imaging at later visits [1]. Significant efforts have been made to improve and standardize training of physicians using diagnostic musculoskeletal ultrasound. These efforts should reduce the variability and improve access to musculoskeletal ultrasound imaging over the coming years.

Sonographic findings have been found to be helpful in distinguishing between mild strains (grade I) and partial tears (grade II) [1]. Distinguish between grade I and II strains with MRI can be challenging as they both will have similar hyperintensity on T2-weighted images [1]. This information is clinically useful as the rehabilitation and management of such injuries differ significantly. Grade I strains tend to have a low risk of tear extension and a quicker return to normal function. While grade II strains typically need a more conservative approach due to increased risk of injury progression and complications. Grade I injuries typically resolve in about 2 weeks, in comparison to the 4 or more weeks of recovery needed for grade II strains.

Because of the superficial nature of the gastrocnemius, ultrasound is particularly useful in imaging injuries to this muscle. The presence of partial tears on ultrasound is seen as focal

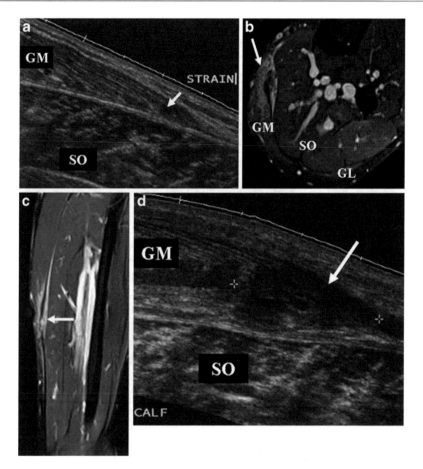

Fig. 7.1 A 27-year-old football player presenting with left calf pain, clinically diagnosed as grade II injury. **a** On ultrasound at initial presentation, a hypoechoic area measuring 1.0 × 0.4 cm was noted *(arrow)*, corresponding with a partial tear of the medial head of the gastrocnemius *(GM)*. Color Doppler imaging was normal (not shown). No evidence of hematoma or other abnormality was observed. Soleus muscle *(SO)* appears intact. Magnetic resonance imaging *(MRI)* was not performed on this patient at this time. **b–d** Follow-up imaging 2 months after initial presentation. **b** Axial and **c** coronal FS T2-w TSE images reveal areas of hyperintensity with feathery appearance, consistent with a partial tear of the medial head of the gastrocnemius muscle with intramuscular edema *(arrow)*. Note the peritendinous edema. **d** On ultrasound, a persistent hypoechogenic area was noted that appeared to have increased in extent *(arrow)*. Color Doppler imaging was normal (not shown). A 7-month follow-up MRI showed complete recovery (not shown). (From [1] ©Springer)

hypoechogenicity of the muscle [1] (Fig. 7.1). In the case of complete tears (grade III), ultrasound can play a role in preoperative assessment if surgery is expected. However, it should be noted that many surgeons are not as familiar or comfortable interpreting ultrasound images and may prefer MRI for surgical planning.

Ultrasound can also be used as a convenient and inexpensive follow-up study for muscle strains. If symptoms have persisted longer than expected or the appropriate return of function has not occurred, a repeat ultrasound can be per-

formed to assess healing and evaluate for complications. Typically, follow-up studies would be performed in 2–3 week intervals as needed.

In addition to assessing muscle injuries, ultrasound has the added benefit of evaluating for the presence of a deep venous thrombosis (DVT) or a ruptured Baker's cyst; two conditions frequently on the differential diagnosis of posterior leg pain and swelling. Moreover, ultrasound can be used for needle guidance in aspiration of fluid collections associated with muscle injuries in the posterior leg [3].

MRI

Magnetic resonance imaging has been standard for imaging muscle injuries for over a decade. MRI is particularly effective in determining the location, severity, and the extent of muscle injuries in the posterior leg. MRI is also useful in assisting the clinician to objectively predict the time required for an athlete to return to their sport with low risk of injury recurrence, to evaluate for possible complications, surgical planning, and to exclude alternative disorders such as stress fracture. MRI is indicated when the clinical diagnosis is uncertain, the patient has an atypical presentation for muscle injury or when a prompt diagnosis is needed to begin the appropriate initial management [5].

A typical MRI protocol uses a combination of T1- and T2-weighted sequences to emphasize the anatomy and any pathologic edema [3] (Fig. 7.2). T1-weighted images highlight fatty structures (fat planes, lipomas, and muscle atrophy), mature myositis ossificans, degenerative tendon conditions, and aid in the characterization of hemorrhagic lesions (hematomas, contusions, hemorrhagic tumors, etc.). Since T2-weighted images are generally fluid sensitive, they are more sensitive to the accumulation of edema in muscle strain injuries and especially useful in a setting of known trauma. It is important to include both short- and long-axis imaging of the leg with a fat- and water-sensitive sequence for each imaging plane. Sagittal and axial images are especially helpful for distinguishing the anterior and posterior aspects of the leg, as the presence of bony structures aid in anatomic reference. A marker can be used on the patient's skin to allow the clinician to correlate clinical symptoms with imaging abnormalities. Contrast is rarely used in evaluation of routine muscle injury but should be included if infection, tumor, or myositis is in the differential.

Acute or sub-acute grade I strains demonstrate bright signal on fluid-sensitive sequences illustrating the edema and hemorrhage at the site of injury. Generally, there is less than 5% involvement of the muscle fibers and a normal appearing myotendinous junction. Grade II strains typically show thinning of the myotendinous junction or muscle fiber disruption in addition to edema and hemorrhage. Grade III strains (high grade or complete tears) show distinct disruption of the muscle-tendon unit with extensive hemorrhage and a wavy appearance of the retracted tendon.

Tennis Leg

"Tennis Leg" is a diagnostic term for muscle injury to the posterior leg. More commonly described today as calf strain, tennis leg has a long and controversial history in the medical literature. It has been described clinically as the sudden onset of sharp pain in the mid-calf during athletics. It most commonly refers to a strain of the medial head of the gastrocnemius and, rarely, the plantaris tendon or soleus muscle. The lack of specificity in the diagnosis of tennis leg stems largely from historical disagreement and the difficulty in being able to differentiate between posterior leg muscle injuries on history and physical exam. Modern imaging and injury classification

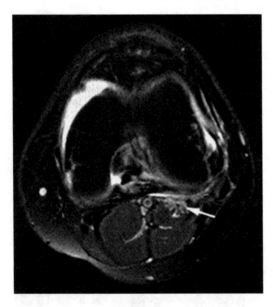

Fig. 7.2 Axial image showing increased fluid signal in the proximal lateral gastrocnemius consistent with a mild strain although the location is somewhat atypical *(arrow)*. (From [3]. Reprinted with permission from Elsevier Limited)

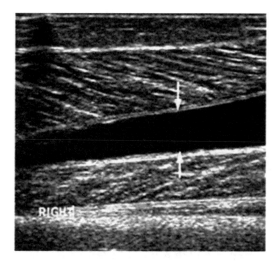

Fig. 7.3 Intermuscular fluid collection between medial gastrocnemius and soleus muscle on ultrasound *(arrows)* in a patient clinically with tennis leg. (From [3]. Reprinted with permission from Elsevier Limited)

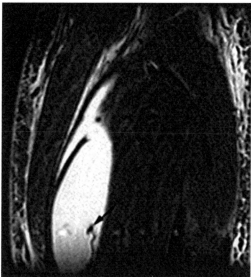

Fig. 7.4 Coronal IR images showing large intermuscular fluid collection between gastrocnemius and soleus muscle as a result of distal plantaris tendon rupture (*arrow* shows retracted tendon). (From [3]. Reprinted with permission from Elsevier Limited)

schemes have made the diagnosis of tennis leg or calf strain antiquated. Should clinical uncertainty about the specificity of the injury exist, both MRI and ultrasound can be used to clarify the location and extent of the injury (Fig. 7.3).

Plantaris Tendon Injury

Injury to the plantaris tendon can clinically mimic a medial head gastrocnemius strain but can be differentiated by imaging. Plantaris tendon ruptures commonly result in an intermuscular fluid collection between the soleus and gastrocnemius with visible retraction of the plantaris muscle appearing as a mass on MRI (8-107) (Fig. 7.4).

Achilles Tendon Injury

Athletes, particularly runners, have a high incidence of Achilles tendon overuse injuries that range from paratendonitis to complete tears [2]. A healthy Achilles tendon appears flat or concave anteriorly except for the focal convexities at the proximal and distal tendon where it is joined with the calf muscles and the calcaneus, respectively.

In tendonitis, the tendon volume increases and becomes oval or round in cross section. The plantaris tendon (present in 90% of people) runs medial to the Achilles tendon prior to its insertion on the calcaneus and should not be mistaken for an Achilles tendon tear, or in the case of a complete tear, not be mistaken for residual intact fibers of the Achilles [2]. MRI or ultrasound can be used to characterize Achilles tendon pathology and diagnosis Achilles tendon tears that are not obvious on physical exam. In a partial tear, fluid signal intensity will be seen within the tendon but can be difficult to distinguish from tendinosis. A tear is more likely if there are findings of edema/hemorrhage surrounding the site of increased signal intensity. The clinician should carefully evaluate any muscle atrophy, underlying tendinosis, and the distance between torn edges of the tendon as each factor will play a role in determining management options. A complete tear will show fiber disruption with a visual gap between the two edges of the retracted tendon. The most common location of Achilles tendon injury is the middle to distal portion and is usually attributed to underlying tendinopathy. Particular attention should also be paid to the insertion site where pain and anterior constriction of the Achilles tendon from a Haglund's deformity can result in tendinopathy. Posterior constriction of the Achilles tendon can occur from direct compression often aggravated by ill-fitting shoes.

Muscle Contusion

Muscle contusions result from direct trauma that causes a series of events that include microscopic rupture and damage to muscle cells, macroscopic defects in the body of the muscle, infiltrative bleeding, and inflammation. These changes tend to occur deep in the muscle and are often less symptomatic than strains. On ultrasound, contusions are described by discontinuity of the normal musculature with indistinct hyperechogenicity that may cross fascial boundaries [1]. In the acute setting, the muscle appears swollen and may be isoechoic with respect to the unaffected adjacent muscle. If there is moderate to severe trauma, disruptions of muscle fibers occur with associated hemorrhage resulting in hematoma formation. Fluid sensitive MRI findings are characterized by hyperintense signal that may have a diffuse appearance with feathery margins. Unlike strains, the location of the contusion is usually not limited to the myotendinous junction and may result in increase in muscle diameter due to the intramuscular hemorrhage and edema. It should be noted that functional recovery from a contusion tends to precede resolution of abnormalities on MRI.

Table 7.1 describes how the typical appearance of new, old, and recurrent injuries differ between ultrasound and MRI.

Baker's or Popliteal Cyst

Baker's or popliteal cysts can be a cause of posterior knee and leg pain. These cysts commonly leak or rupture causing pain and swelling in the calf. Clinically, a ruptured Baker's cyst can be difficult to distinguish from other common causes of posterior leg pain such as gastrocnemius strains or DVT. Ultrasound and MRI are typically used in the initial workup of suspected Baker's cyst rupture if uncertainty remains after clinical evaluation. Ultrasonography can be used to localize the cyst and visualize the extent of local edema as well as differentiate between muscle strains, popliteal aneurysms, DVT, or other popliteal masses. Radiographs have limited benefit for viewing the cyst itself but will pick up bony or calcific abnormalities that can be associated with the cyst.

Delayed Onset Muscle Soreness (DOMS)

This clinical entity refers to delayed muscle pain and soreness following a large increase in recent exertion. The diagnosis of delayed onset muscle soreness (DOMS) can often be made by the history and exam alone. MRI can be diagnostic and may generally shows a similar signal intensity pattern seen in grade I muscle strain. However, the changes associated with DOMS are generally more diffuse and typically affect more than one muscle and/or compartment of the leg. Ultrasound may be normal or show hyperechogenicity in several muscles.

Muscle Herniation

Muscle herniations are an uncommon but significant cause of posterior leg pain. These injuries typically occur after traumatic injury to the leg that results in a focal area of fascia disruption. The underlying muscle then herniates through this defect causing focal pain, swelling, and dysfunction with activity. The diagnosis of muscle herniation is often best determined clinically but if uncertainty remains regarding the diagnosis, MRI and US can be used for confirmation. The muscle will appear as a focal protrusion through a fascial defect on both imaging modalities but the findings can be subtle. For this reason, dynamic imaging during muscle contraction should be considered to make the herniation more pronounced aiding in diagnosis [3, 6].

Table 7.1 Differentiation between new, old, and recurrent injuries by imaging. (From [1]. ©Springer)

Type of injury	Imaging findings	
	MR imaging	Ultrasound
New (acute)		
Grade I strain	Intramuscular "feathery" hyperintensity on fluid-sensitive sequences without muscle fiber disruption	Areas of intramuscular hyperechogenicity and perifascial hypoechogenicity (fluid collection)
Grade II strain	Hyperintensity (edema and hemorrhage) intramuscularly or at the MTJ, with extension along the fascial planes between muscle groups	Discontinuity of muscle fibers with hypervascularity around disrupted muscle fibers
	Irregularity and mild laxity of tendon fibers	Altered echogenicity and loss of perimysial striation adjacent to the MTJ
	Hematoma at the MTJ is pathognomonic	Intramuscular fluid collection (hypoechogenicity) with a surrounding hyperechoic halo
		Complete discontinuity of muscle fibers associated with extensive edema and hematoma, and possible retraction of tendon
Grade III strain	Complete discontinuity of muscle fibers associated with extensive edema and hematoma, and possible retraction of tendon	Ill-defined area of hyperechogenicity in the muscle, which may cross fascial planes
Contusion	T1-weighted and fluid-sensitive sequences may show hypo to hyperintensity	
Hematoma	Acute (<48 h): typically isointense to muscles on T1-weighted images	Appears as a hypoechoic fluid collection and may contain debris
	Sub-acute (<30 days): higher signal intensity than muscle on both T1-weighted and fluid-sensitive sequences; variable signal intensities within hematoma	Variable appearance (anechoic, hypoechoic, or hyperechoic) within 24 h of injury; appearance changes over the next few days becoming hypoechoic or anechoic
Avulsion	Redundant tendon edge lying within large fluid collection/hematoma	Evaluation is difficult due to the presence of mixed echogenicity hematoma with similar echogenicity to the avulsed tendon
	A small bony fragment	
Old (chronic)		
Muscle enlargement or atrophy	Chronic avulsion has no surrounding fluid and tendon edges may be difficult to define	
Scar tissue morphological	Scar tissue appears hypointense on all pulse sequences	Areas of scar tissue have irregular features and display heterogeneous echo texture
Chronic hematoma	Dark signal intensity rim seen on all pulse sequences due to hemosiderin (chronic hematoma)	

MTJ musculotendinous junction

Myositis Ossificans

The diagnosis of myositis ossificans can be difficult. Traditionally, plain radiographs or CT were thought to be sufficient for diagnosis but abnormalities are typically not visible until mature ossification occurs several weeks after the injury [7].

During acute to sub-acute stage, MRI can pick up what is known as the zone phenomenon on T-2 weighted imaging, which is an intramuscular mass with a central area of slight hyperintensity surrounded by inflammatory tissue edema. Early US will show these three concentric layers as well: a hypoechoic peripheral layer surrounding a thin hyperechoic layer corresponding to the ossification, and a hypoechoic zone in the center [7]. Later on in the course, the pathognomonic ossification surrounding a clear area, apart from adjacent bony areas, will appear on X-ray.

Stress Fractures—Tibia and Fibula

Stress injuries and fractures are a common cause of leg pain in athletes. Stress fractures are caused by repetitive activities and often occur in the setting of increased intensity or volume of weight-bearing activity. The range of stress-related injuries in the leg includes periosteal reaction, stress fractures, and displaced fractures. Tibial stress injuries represent the vast majority of stress injuries in the leg. This corresponds to the dominant biomechanical role of the tibia in weight bearing.

Stress injuries of the leg usually present as the insidious onset of focal exertional leg pain. Stress injuries are usually associated with recent changes in activity, ground surface, gait, or footwear. Examination finding can be subtle but usually include bony tenderness at the site of injury and localized swelling. Loading or tension of the affected bone will typically reproduce symptoms.

Although often negative in the acute setting, plain X-rays of the tibia and fibula should be ordered in patients with suspected stress injury of the leg. Indications of stress injury on plain films include periosteal reaction, focal sclerosis, cortical thickening, or frank disruption of the cortex. Cortical disruption is typically lucent, linear, transverse, and focal.

If plain radiographs confirm stress injury, no further imaging is usually needed. However, if plain films are negative and clinical suspicion for stress fracture remains then either X-rays should be repeated in several weeks or advanced imaging can be ordered for further evaluation. Triple phase bone scan, single photon emission computed tomography (SPECT), or MRI are standard imaging options for radiographic negative stress injuries. Bone scan has excellent sensitivity, but lacks the specificity of MRI and SPECT imaging. Bone scans may not be positive in acute

setting and may show persistent abnormal bone metabolism even after clinical resolution of the injury. In addition, bone scan can be limited in the detection of minute localized abnormalities. SPECT imaging can improve the sensitivity and specificity of traditional bone scans. Unlike a traditional bone scan, SPECT scans obtain multiple projections from the gamma camera which are then reconstructed to improve contrast resolution. SPECT imaging can be integrated with CT scanning (SPECT/CT) to precisely correlate the functional imaging of SPECT with the high resolution structural imaging of CT. MRI has both excellent sensitivity and specificity for stress injuries. MRI can detect early stress-related changes and can also provide additional information regarding soft tissue injuries in the differential for stress injuries of the leg. For these reasons MRI imaging is often the imaging modality of choice for radiographic negative bone injuries [6].

Nervous System Disorders

Electrodiagnostics (EDx), which include electromyography (EMG) and nerve conduction studies (NCS), are used to evaluate suspected impairments of the peripheral nervous system. They are an extension of the physical exam for the electrodiagnostic medicine consultant and aid in differentiating neurogenic versus non-neurogenic causes of pain, weakness, and paresthesias. A broad differential of causes can present with these symptoms including lumbar radiculopathy, focal nerve entrapment, peripheral neuropathy, and vascular concerns. Like imaging, EMG together with NCS can aid the clinician in diagnosing the precise anatomic location and reveal the underlying pathology of the presenting complaint. EDx testing is specific but lacks sensitivity in diagnosing acute or intermittent nerve injury. For this reason, patients with intermittent symptoms or with symptoms of less than 3 weeks duration are unlikely to benefit from EDx. However, when EDx is positive it helps rule in the location of a peripheral nerve lesion and assess the degree of nerve damage; both of which guide management options.

Compressive lesions or trauma to the nerve can cause focal entrapment neuropathies, which result in demyelination or axonal loss of sensory and/or motor nerves. In the case of compressive entrapment syndromes, sensory nerves are frequently affected more severely and earlier when compared to motor nerves. Common culprits in the setting of entrapment in the leg include the common peroneal nerve at the head of the fibula, deep peroneal nerve in the anterior ankle, superficial peroneal nerve where it penetrates the deep fascia 10–13 cm proximal to the lateral malleolus, and the tibial nerve in the popliteal fossa.

Vascular Disorders

The differential of posterior leg and calf pain involves several vascular disorders including: venous thrombosis, thrombophlebitis, peripheral artery disease, popliteal artery entrapment syndrome (PAES), and cystic adventitial disease. Cystic adventitial disease is a rare vascular obstructive condition that typically affects the popliteal artery. It is most common in young men, and like other arterial vascular disorders presents as claudication. Venous thrombosis and thrombophlebitis are common and typically present as calf pain, tenderness, and swelling. DVT can lead to pulmonary embolism or the post-thrombotic syndrome. Post-thrombotic syndrome is typified by chronic leg pain and edema, skin changes, and venous stasis ulcers. The work up of vascular leg pain can include duplex ultrasound, ankle brachial index, and potentially MRI or CT angiography for PAES and cystic adventitial disease.

Duplex ultrasound can image the vessels and measure blood flow. A duplex ultrasound can be done of both the veins and the arteries. A duplex venous ultrasound is the standard test used to evaluate the leg for venous thrombosis. It can determine the extent and specific location of the thrombosis. An ankle brachial index measures and compares blood pressure in the arm and leg to assess for arterial disease. Ankle brachial pressures can be done at rest or before and after ex-

ercise. CT angiography can be used to confirm static or dynamic limitations to blood flow. Magnetic resonance angiography (MRA) can be used to visualize the vascular system and detect structural lesions or flow limitations.

Chronic Exertional Compartment Syndrome (CECS)

Chronic exertional compartment syndrome (CECS)-related leg pain is thought to be caused by reversible ischemia of the involved compartment of the leg. Intracompartmental pressure and demand for oxygenated blood rises with exertion. As the pressure within the compartment approaches the blood pressure, a mismatch occurs between the availability and demand for oxygenated blood to the muscles within the compartment. The resulting ischemia and increased compartment pressure causes pain and dysfunction of the structures within the compartment.

The diagnosis of CECS is made by directly measuring intracompartmental pressures in a patient with a suggestive history and physical exam. Commonly accepted values include ≥ 15-mmHg pre-exercise, ≥ 30-mmHg 1-min post exercise, or ≥ 20-mmHg 5-min post exercise. Although direct measurement of compartment pressure remains the gold standard for diagnosing compartment syndrome, MRI and near infrared spectroscopy of oxygen saturation have also been used for diagnosis by visualizing the ischemic changes associated with CECS.

Laboratory Tests

There are a vast number of laboratory tests that can be ordered in the work up of posterior leg pain. Most of these investigations should be performed only for specific clinical concerns and not as a routine workup for posterior leg pain. Tests that can assist the clinician in narrowing the differential diagnosis of posterior leg pain include but are not limited to: plasma muscle enzymes (creatinine kinase, aldolase, lactate dehydrogenase, and aminotransferases) for suspected myopathy or muscular dystrophy, and serologic tests when concerned for inflammatory myopathy or associated connective tissue diseases. When evaluating for suspected myopathy without a clear diagnosis after the history, physical examination, and laboratory, radiologic, and electromyographic evaluations, a muscle biopsy should be considered. Other tests could include a complete blood count and metabolic profile, creatinine kinase, and myoglobin for infectious etiologies and rhabdomyolysis.

Conclusions

Clinicians who dedicate a large part of their practice to musculoskeletal injuries have a significant amount of pressure to accurately diagnose, manage, and quantify the prognosis of sports injuries. Imaging can play a vital role in assisting the clinician to determine recurrence risks, management options, and the amount of time needed to safely return to play. The imaging modalities described in this chapter should not be used independently, but in conjunction with a thorough history and physical examination as well as other ancillary tests. Imaging during the rehabilitation of the injury can be used to monitor the healing process and used together with clinical symptoms to guide therapeutic decisions.

Future areas of clinically important advancement in musculoskeletal imaging include long tract MRI of nerves and further elucidating the role of imaging during the rehabilitation phase of muscle injuries. The role of musculoskeletal ultrasound imaging will likely continue to grow and evolve [8]. Technological developments and evidence-based imaging protocols offer the promise of less expensive yet effective imaging techniques to reduce overall morbidity and costs associated with musculoskeletal injuries.

References

1. Hayashi D, Hamilton B, Guermazi A, De villiers R, Crema MD, Roemer FW. Traumatic injuries of thigh and calf muscles in athletes: role and clinical relevance of MR imaging and ultrasound. Insights Imaging. 2012;3(6):591–601.
2. Bresler M, Mar W, Toman J. Diagnostic imaging in the evaluation of leg pain in athletes. Clin Sports Med. 2012;31(2):217–45.
3. Armfield DR, Kim DH, Towers JD, Bradley JP, Robertson DD. Sports-related muscle injury in the lower extremity. Clin Sports Med. 2006;25(4):803–42.
4. Bryan Dixon J. Gastrocnemius vs. soleus strain: how to differentiate and deal with calf muscle injuries. Curr Rev Musculoskelet Med. 2009;2(2):74–7.
5. Pedowitz R, Chung CB, Resnick D. Magnetic Resonance imaging in orthopedic sports medicine. New York: Springer Science & Business Media; 2008:1–20.
6. David TS. Missed Lower extremity and spine fractures in athletes. Curr Sports Med Rep. 2003;2:295–302.
7. Lacout A, Jarraya M, Marcy P-Y, Thariat J, Carlier RY. Myositis ossificans imaging: keys to successful diagnosis. The Indian J Radiol Imaging. 2012;22(1):35–9. doi:10.4103/0971-3026.95402.
8. Borg-stein J, Zaremski JL, Hanford MA. New concepts in the assessment and treatment of regional musculoskeletal pain and sports injury. PM R. 2009;1(8):744–54.
9. Breitenseher MMR. Imaging strategies for the lower extremities. New York: Thieme; 2005.
10. Martinoli C. Musculoskeletal ultrasound: technical guidelines. Insights Imaging. 2010;1(3):99–141.
11. Roy PC. Electrodiagnostic evaluation of lower extremity neurogenic problems. Foot Ankle Clin. 2011;16(2):225–42.
12. Mitchell AW, Lee JC, Healy JC. The use of ultrasound in the assessment and treatment of Achilles tendinosis. J Bone Joint Surg Br. 2009;91(11):1405–9.
13. Lee JC, Mitchell AWM, Healy JC. Imaging of muscle injury in the elite athlete. Br J Radiol. 2012;85(1016):1173–85. doi:10.1259/bjr/84622172.
14. Bergmann G, et al. Gastrocnemius muscle herniation as a rare differential diagnosis of ankle sprain: case report and review of the literature. Patient Saf Surg. 2012;6:5.

Part III

Treatment of Muscular Injuries in the Posterior Leg

Acute Injuries in the Posterior Leg

Stephen M. Simons and Jeremy L. Riehm

Introduction

To understand the treatment principles of muscular injuries in the posterior leg, the clinician must have a firm understanding of the structural anatomy and pathophysiology as discussed in Part I. Knowledge of these fundamentals will allow for optimal patient outcomes and serve as a guide during the workup of muscular injury. To assure successful treatment, the clinician must also feel comfortable with the steps in ascertaining a proper diagnosis as discussed in Part II. A correct diagnosis is crucial as there are severe long-term complications that can ensue from an improperly diagnosed muscular injury. Part III discusses treatment of muscular injuries in the posterior leg and starts with this chapter on acute injuries.

The posterior leg musculature can sustain various acute injuries such as contusions, muscular strains or tears, frank rupture, and puncture wounds. Many of these injuries, predominately strains, may present late and consequently will be managed by the clinician while in the sub-acute or even chronic stage. Sub-acute and chronic injuries are discussed in detail in Chap. 9. The acute management of muscle injuries refers to the time immediately following the injury and the following several days (see Fig. 9.1 in Chap. 9).

After the sustaining muscular injury, there is an inflammatory cascade which initiates the healing process. These inflammatory changes define the acute phase (see Table 4.1 in Chap. 4). This differentiates acute injures from sub-acute and chronic injuries when proliferation and remodeling of soft tissue dominate healing [1]. Details of these inflammatory mediators and their sequela are discussed in detail in Chap. 4. The mechanism of injury most often involves a history of a traumatic event. Occasionally, muscular strains and some other acute injuries may occur without a clearly described inciting event.

Acute muscular injuries to the posterior leg are generally treated conservatively. The goal of treatment is to restore the muscle to normal structure and function. Surgery is rarely required to achieve these goals, as many conditions are amenable to an array of less invasive measures. Notable exceptions include complete ruptures and the development of acute compartment syndrome, the surgical management of which is discussed in Chap. 10. This chapter will first discuss contusions in detail, followed by the spectrum of other acute injuries. Table 8.1 summarizes the treatment methods for acute muscular injuries in the posterior leg.

S. M. Simons (✉)
Sports Medicine, Saint Joseph Regional Medical Center, Mishawaka, IN, USA
e-mail: simonss@sjrmc.com

J. L. Riehm
Medical Education, Saint Joseph Regional Medical Center, Mishawaka, IN, USA
e-mail: jeremyriehm@gmail.com

Table 8.1 Summary of the treatment methods for acute muscular injuries in the lower leg

Injury	Treatment
Contusion	RICE, NSAIDs, and early range of motion and rehabilitation
	Prevention and management of myositis ossificans
	Consider immobilization in tension to limit hematoma formation
Strain/tear	RICE, NSAIDs, and early range of motion and rehabilitation
	Partial weight bearing
	Consider heel wedges
Rupture	RICE, NSAIDs, and early range of motion and rehabilitation
	Partial weight bearing
	Consider heel wedges
	Consider surgery if complete loss of function
Acute compartment syndrome	Emergent fasciotomy
Stab/puncture wounds	Irrigation +/− debridement +/− tetanus and/or antibiotic prophylaxis

RICE rest, ice, compression, and elevation, *NSAIDs* nonsteroidal anti-inflammatory drugs

Contusions

Contusions occur by direct or sheer forces applied to the muscle resulting in capillary and venous disruption that causes an intramuscular damage and hematoma. The injury promptly creates a cascade of pathophysiologic changes followed by immediate healing efforts. The acute management strategy focuses on limiting the extent of the hematoma formation. Proper treatment is necessary to avoid potential complications such as compartment syndrome or myositis ossificans.

Rest, ice, compression, and elevation (RICE) principles apply to acute contusion injury. The use of these four principles is recommended because they promote reduction of inflammation and swelling. Resting (relative immobilization) a contusion injury will help prevent further hematoma formation and therefore limit the extent of blood that needs to be reabsorbed and associated changes to the muscle and soft tissue. There is evidence to support immediate muscle immobilization to help limit hematoma formation [2, 3]. Specifically, immobilization while maintaining some muscle tension is suggested. A West Point study investigated a protocol for treating quadriceps contusion. This study found significantly shorter length of disability using an initial treatment protocol that placed the quadriceps on tension by holding the extremity in a knee flexed/hip extended position [3]. Reminiscent of immediate

management of quadriceps contusion, resting the gastrocnemius in tension—foot dorsiflexed and knee extended—will theoretically provide an intrinsic tamponade effect by the enveloping fascia. Placing the gastrocnemius in tension will not only limit swelling and hemorrhage but will also minimize scar formation and preserve elasticity, contractility, and strength [3]. While there are no available studies specific to the lower leg, using the data presented in the West Point quadriceps protocol, one can infer that using such a regimen for the gastrocnemius would lead to subsequent accelerated rehabilitation and an ability to achieve full ankle dorsiflexion more rapidly.

While brief immobilization can provide therapeutic benefits as described above, prolonged immobilization is associated with longer periods of disability. Mobilization of the muscle leads to regeneration of its components and restoration of biomechanical strength. It is not possible to reliably determine when immobilization should end, and mobilizations begin since repetitive activation of the muscle too early may incite further connective tissue damage and scarring. The literature suggests that when the hematoma is stable, early restoration of motion can begin as long as the patient is comfortable and pain free at rest. Pain-free or minimally uncomfortable passive range of motion is introduced early and followed by a gradual progression to active range of motion [3].

Ice (cryotherapy) facilitates therapeutic effects on acute soft tissue injuries by decreasing pain and muscle spasm and also limiting inflammation via vasoconstriction mechanisms. This vascular constriction to local tissue reduces reactive hyperemia from the injury and incudes leukocyte recruitment. Using ice for soft tissue injury has long been employed and is a mainstay of acute injury management. However, there is very little consensus regarding the most effective duration, frequency, or mode of application of cryotherapy treatments. The clinician should advise the patient to limit direct contact of cryotherapy treatments to the skin due to possible incidental damage to the soft tissues and give caution regarding signs of frostbite [4–6].

Compression limits local blood flow and can prevent progression of hematoma formation. The literature suggests that the combination of compression and cryotherapy may be more beneficial than either modality used alone. Lastly, elevation takes advantage of gravity and hydrostatic pressure to limit extravasation and thereby reduces edema [6].

Aspiration of hematomas or other fluid collections associated with the contusion should be considered in the acute period. The decision to aspirate is based on the location, extent, and patient factors. Any attempt at aspiration has risks of introducing contamination into the effected tissue and limiting the local tamponade effect. Surgical evacuation of a large hematoma can be considered but is typically deferred unless complications such as acute compartment syndrome are manifest.

During the rehabilitation process, care is necessary to avoid reinjury. Myositis ossificans can develop following the primary injury, however, a reinjured muscle further risks developing this significant complication [2]. Myositis ossificans is a debilitating condition of extra-skeletal ossification of the injured muscle or other soft tissue. Sometimes, the calcifications spontaneously reabsorb and the condition may go unrecognized. Surgical debridement may become necessary if myositis ossificans remains symptomatic and unresponsive to conservative measures such as indomethacin [2].

Use of nonsteroidal anti-inflammatory drugs (NSAIDs) in the setting of muscle contusion is controversial. Given the platelet inhibition effect, NSAIDs may worsen hematoma formation. A safer option may be to use simple analgesics such as acetaminophen. However, a controlled animal study showed that utilization of acetaminophen versus the NSAIDs had similar effects on muscle healing [7]. Conversely, early use of NSAIDs may avert risk of developing myositis ossificans. Evidence for this use is inferred from studies showing a decrease in heterotopic bone formation after total hip replacement in patients receiving indomethacin [8]. Since there are no available randomized controlled studies regarding utilization and timing of various analgesics, the clinician must weigh the risks and benefits when implementing these medications. To supplement the treatment of contusions, one may direct ancillary staff to employ the use of therapeutic ultrasound. It should be noted that although therapeutic ultrasound is commonly used during rehabilitation, it does not appear to effect the regeneration of skeletal muscle following contusion [9].

Stab or Puncture Wounds

Acute penetrating trauma from stab or puncture wounds can cause muscular injures in the posterior leg. The focus of treatment for stab or puncture wounds is generally aimed at reducing risk of infection. Thorough irrigation and cleansing of the wound should be performed. The clinician should determine the need for any tissue debridement or surgical repair. Surgical debridement is needed when there is deep tissue involvement and severe contamination. When indicated, tetanus and/or antibiotic prophylaxis should be used [1].

Strain, Tear, and Rupture

Most other acute injuries to the posterior leg fall in the spectrum of rupture, tear, and strain. Excessive tensile forces lead to overstraining of the individual myofibers. The severity of injury is

Table 8.2 Three-part classification system for grading of calf injuries. (From [7]. ©J. Bryan Dixon)

Grade	Symptoms	Signs	Pathologic correlation	Radiology correlation
Grade 1 First degree—mild	Sharp pain at the time of injury or pain with activity. Usually able to continue activity	Mild pain and localized tenderness. Mild spasm and swelling. No or minimal loss of strength and ROM	<10% muscle fiber disruption	Bright signal on fluid-sensitive sequences. Feathery appearance. <5% muscle fiber involvement
Grade 2 Second degree—moderate	Unable to continue activity	Clear loss of strength and ROM	>10–50% disruption of muscle fibers	Change in myotendinous junction. Edema and hemorrhage
Grade 3 Third degree—severe	Immediate severe pain, disability	Complete loss of muscle function. Palpable defect or mass. Possible positive Thompson test	50–100% disruption of muscle fibers	Complete disruption of discontinuity of muscle. Extensive edema and hemorrhage. Wavy tendon morphology and retraction

ROM range of motion

determined by the amount of force and the ability of the soft tissue to withstand tension. Ruptures involve complete dissociation of muscle fibers, while tears are generally considered partial disruption in the contractile tissue. Strains are simply due to an overstretching of the muscle fibers with no disruption. As discussed in Part II, the clinician can use a combination of physical exam and imaging to assist in diagnosis of calf injuries. Grading calf injuries is typically quantitated on a 1–3 severity scale (Table 8.2).

The muscles of the superficial posterior compartment consist of the triceps surae (gastrocnemius, soleus, and plantaris) commonly referred to as the "calf muscle." The plantaris is a vestigial muscle that is present only in 15% of the population. This muscle is frequently injured concurrently with the gastrocnemius and soleus. There have been only a few case reports of isolated plantaris injuries and treatment methods are similar to other calf injuries. The caveat to these plantaris injuries is that they very closely mimic the typical clinical presentation of acute deep venous thrombosis. There is a paucity of literature available regarding treatment of acute muscular strain or rupture in the deep posterior compartment. Injuries to these muscles most always presents as a chronic or occasionally sub-acute condition [1].

Gastrocnemius and Soleus

The gastrocnemius is the most commonly injured muscle in the posterior lower leg and most of the available literature comes from the studies on this muscle. The gastroc is more prone to rupture due to the characteristic biarticular anatomy and muscle fiber composition with fast-twitch fibers (see Table 4.1 in Chap. 4; [7, 10]). Acute gastrocnemius muscle injuries occur when the muscle experiences a sudden acceleration upon a dorsiflexed ankle position such as the one commonly seen on the tennis court. Another common mechanism is a sudden eccentric load into ankle dorsiflexion, as seen in the case of a snowboarder making a hard landing. The gastrocnemius's musculotendinous junction and its medial belly are most commonly injured [11]. This injury to the medial gastroachilles junction is commonly referred to as "tennis leg." However, "tennis leg" is frequently regarded as a misnomer as there are many injury mechanisms that occur off the tennis court. Other muscles of the posterior lower leg are injured by various mechanisms. As discussed in the case of gastrocnemius muscle, the vectors involved during the injury will determine which structures are affected.

The gastrocnemius and soleus have some important distinctions and therefore must be discussed in further detail. While the gastrocnemius and soleus are frequently injured concomitantly, it is important to distinguish the two injuries if possible. Isolation of either injury can be performed by clinical examination. By placing the knee into full knee flexion or extension, the examiner can manipulate the role of the gastrocnemius in movement of the ankle. The gastrocnemius is the primary muscle responsible for ankle plantarflexion when the knee is placed into complete extension. When the knee is in full flexion, the soleus is primarily responsible for plantarflexion. The rehabilitation potential is significantly greater if isolated injuries can be accurately diagnosed. The ability to utilize dorsiflexion and plantarflexion at the ankle while isolating a particular muscle simply by flexing or extending the knee allows for specific muscle rehabilitation.

Generally, nonoperative care is the standard for gastrocnemius strain injuries. In rare cases, surgery may be offered if the rupture is substantial and results in complete loss of muscle function. Although surgical repair of the musculotendinous junction can be offered, the literature does not support a distinguishing favorable outcome over standard nonoperative care. Although nonoperative management or watchful waiting is the principle strategy for these strain injuries, the clinician needs to be alert to the possibility of acute compartment syndromes necessitating early surgical intervention [11].

Without symptoms of acute compartment syndrome, the treatment regimen of muscular strain, tear, or rupture most always involves a wide array of conservative measures. Early treatment protocols utilize RICE therapy and partial weight bearing and NSAIDs. Additionally, early ankle motion is instituted. Careful implementation regarding timing of NSAIDs must still be considered as discussed in the section on muscle contusions. Many patients will develop ecchymosis in the days following the injury and the patient should be assured regarding this normal process.

Individuals who have severe strains may require crutches, though some clinicians have opted to use rocker-bottom postoperative boots instead. Bilateral 1-in. heel wedges are helpful

if the patient is able to ambulate. Gentle stretching may be initiated as soon as it can be accomplished without pain and stretches held for at least 15 s may reduce scar tissue and facilitate healing [8, 12]. Additionally, strengthening may commence as soon as 24 h after initial injury. Muscle strength should be recovered through a program of controlled eccentric and concentric lifting. Massage is also helpful as an adjunct to strengthening [8]. Recently, autologous plateletrich plasma (PRP) has been shown to shorten recovery time after a muscle strain injury [13].

Return to training and competition generally can occur after 4–6 weeks, although severe tears may take up to 12 weeks to heal. Full participation in sports is permitted when strength is nearly equal to unaffected leg and symptoms have resolved. If rehabilitation of an acute gastrocnemius injury is inadequate, weak scar tissue may become injured repeatedly resulting in chronic strain. Podiatric and gait assessment may be indicated to correct biomechanical factors that contribute to calf tightness and slow recovery [11].

Acute Compartment Syndrome

The clinician needs to be alert to the possible complication of acute compartment syndrome in the setting of muscular injuries to the posterior leg. The posterior compartments of the leg (superficial and deep) are a confined space. Swelling within the compartment can lead to compression of the neurovascular structures and muscle resulting in tissue necrosis. Acute compartment syndrome necessitates urgent compartment fasciotomy which relieves compression on the muscle and neurovascular structures [11].

The diagnosis of acute compartment syndrome is made by clinical examination or direct compartment pressure testing. The clinical signs and symptoms of acute compartment syndrome include the "5 Ps" of compartment syndrome: pain, pallor, paresthesias, paralysis, and pulselessness. The involved compartment will exhibit swelling and firmness on palpation; passive range of motion of the distal extremity is also often present. In addition, complaints of pain out of proportion to the trauma event and pain not responsive to medications suggest compartment syndrome.

Ps of Compartment Syndrome
- Pain
  - out of proportion
  - unresponsive to treatment
  - with passive range of motion of the toes
- Pallor (late finding)
- Paresthesias (late finding)
- Paralysis (late finding)
- Pulselessness (late finding)
- Palpable swelling and firmness

If the history and physical examination are suggestive but not conclusive for acute compartment syndrome, then direct measurement of compartment pressure is indicated. Compartment pressure of 35 mmHg or within 30 mmHg of the diastolic blood pressure is consistent with the diagnosis.

References

1. Tero AH, Teppo LN, Minna K, Hannu K, Markku J. Muscle injuries. Am J of Sports Med. 2005;33(5):745–61.
2. Beiner JM, Jokl P. Muscle contusion injury and myositis ossificans traumatica. Clin Orthop Relat Res. 2002;403:S110–9.
3. Ryan JB, Wheeler JH, Hopkinson WJ, Arciero RA, Kolakowski KR. Quadraceps contusions. West point update. Am J Sports Med. 1991;16:299–304.
4. Bleakley C, McDonough S, DacAuley D. The use of ice in the treatment of acute soft-tissue injury. Am J Med. 2004;32(1):251–61.
5. Lee H, Natsui H, Akimoto T, Yanag K, Ohshima N, Kono I. Effects of cryotherapy after contusion using real-time intravital microscopy. Med Sci Sports Exerc. 2005;37(7):1093–8.
6. Schaser K, Disch AC, Stover JF, Lauffer A, Bail HJ, Mittlmeier T. Prolonged superficial local cryotherapy attenuates microcirculatory impairment, regional inflammation, and muscle necrosis after closed soft tissue injury in rats. Am J of Sports Med. 2007;35(1):93–1028.
7. Dixon BJ. Gastrocnemius vs. soleus strain: how to differentiate and deal with calf muscle injuries. Curr Rev Musculoskelet Med. 2009;2(2):74–7. (Published online 2009 May 23).
8. Fijn R, Koorevaar RT, Brouwers RBJ. Prevention of heterotopic ossification after total hip replacement with NSAIDs. Pharm World Sci. 2003;25:138–45.
9. Wilkin LD, Merrick, MA, Kirby TE, Devor ST. Influence of therapeutic ultrasound on skeletal muscle regeneration following blunt contusion. Int J Sports Med. 2004;25:73–7.
10. Armfield DR, Kim DH, Towers JD, Bradley JP, Roberson DD. Sports-related muscle injury in the lower extremity. Clin Sports Med. 2006;25(4):803–42.
11. Glazer JL, Hosey RG. Soft-tissue injuries of the lower extremity. Prim Care. 2004;31(4):1005–2.
12. Roberts JM, Wilson K. Effect of stretching duration on active and passive range of motion in the lower extremity. Br J Sports Med. 1999;33:259–63.
13. Hammond JW, Hinton RY, Curl LA, Muriel JM, LoveringRM. Use of autologous platelet-rich plasma to treat muscle strain injuries. Am J Sports Med. 2009;37(6):1135–42.

Sub-acute and Chronic Injuries in the Posterior Leg

9

Stephen M. Simons and Christopher C. Jordan

Introduction

Defining Sub-acute

Before a discussion can take place regarding treatment of sub-acute injuries, a definition of "sub-acute" must be clarified. Generally speaking, sub-acute implies the spectrum of injury between acute and chronic. However, this determination is often based on phases of soft tissue healing. Soft tissue healing is divided into the inflammatory phase, proliferative phase, and maturation phase. These correlate closely to the acute, sub-acute, and chronic phases of injury, respectively. Therefore, the sub-acute phase of healing begins around 3–4 days and can last up to 21–28 days or longer [1, 2] (Fig. 9.1). The emphasis during this sub-acute phase is on repair and regeneration of injured tissue. It is important to determine what types of physiologic changes take place during this time in order to adequately examine treatment goals as well as available medications and modalities that are aimed at recovery for the various lower extremity injuries to be discussed throughout this chapter.

During the sub-acute phase, growth and regeneration take place primarily through angiogenesis intermixed with collagen formation. This is stimulated by multiple growth factors including vascular endothelial growth factor (VEGF), platelet derived growth factor (PDGF), and fibroblast growth factor (FGF; Table 9.1). While this process is an integral part to overall healing, it can also result in scar tissue formation or prolong the overall healing process [1, 3]. Therapies should be aimed at reducing such effects while maximizing the benefits of the sub-acute phase of healing.

Defining Chronic

Chronic injury can be defined both quantitatively and histologically. These injuries involve a prolonged course of repair and regeneration when compared to sub-acute injury. This consists of continued satellite cell differentiation, type I collagen production, and fibroblast proliferation [4]. Typically, chronic injuries are the result of maladaptive patterns of regeneration and repair resulting in persistent inflammation and decreased function [5]. This can be exacerbated by severity of injury, overuse, or premature return to previous level of activity. For those interested in additional detail on the pathophysiology of skeletal muscle injury and the phases of healing, an extensive review can be found in Chap. 4.

S. M. Simons (✉) · C. C. Jordan
Sports Medicine, Saint Joseph Regional Medical Center, Mishawaka, IN 46545, USA
e-mail: simonss@sjrmc.com

C. C. Jordan
e-mail: jordanc@sjrmc.com

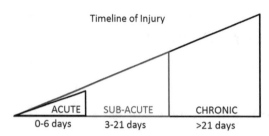

Fig. 9.1 Approximate phases of healing. *Acute* (0–6 days), *sub-acute* (3–21 days), and *chronic* (>21 days)

Gastrocnemius

Gastrocnemius muscle injuries occur most frequently in middle-aged or older adults, although these injuries will also afflict younger athletes. Most vulnerable are those who participate in one of the following sports: running, basketball, football, skiing, and racquet sports [6]. Biomechanically, the most common mechanism of injury is caused by a sudden knee extension while the foot is already dorsiflexed [7, 8]. The location of injury within the gastrocnemius is primarily the medial head at the myotendinous junction (MTJ). This region is considered the weakest part of the muscle–tendon complex [9]. The medial head also has a prolonged attachment, which may provide stronger forces than the lateral head of the gastrocnemius [8].

Most sub-acute gastrocnemius strains will be evident by history and physical exam. Patients will usually recall a single event antecedent to symptom onset, although occasionally, the event is either forgotten or was overshadowed by distracting events such as sport participation. When prompted, the patient may be able to localize the site of pain at onset to the medial calf, or they may report vague posterior leg pain.

Examination sequence is similar to other orthopedic injuries: inspect for swelling, ecchymosis, or deformity. The examiner should then palpate carefully for a single or broad-based tender location. A palpable defect should be sought as well. The novice must be cautioned, as sometimes a normal myotendinous junction may be interpreted as being defective. Examining the contralateral leg can provide comparison. The examiner may also ask the patient to provide a plantar flexion force against resistance (i.e., the examiner's hand) to elicit pain or a noticeable defect. Inspection and palpation can also be performed with the patient standing, followed by heel-rise efforts if tolerated.

Imaging typically is not required to make the diagnosis. However, the elite athlete may benefit from magnetic resonance imaging (MRI) or ultrasound examination to gain additional information on prognosis and healing. Imaging is also useful to help exclude other causes of calf pain, which include thrombophlebitis, compartment syndrome, ruptured popliteal cyst, or plantaris rupture [8]. Diffuse swelling to the lower leg may also prompt the clinician to consider deep vein thrombosis (DVT). If diagnostic imaging is needed, the two primary methods include MRI and ultrasound; however, MRI is preferred for sub-acute injuries due to increased visibility of muscle injuries [8]. In particular, T1-weighted images are beneficial in the assessment of sub-acute hemorrhage associated with gastrocnemius strains [8]. MRI is also superior to ultrasound

Table 9.1 Function of growth factors involved in sub-acute healing phase

Growth factor	Functions
VEGF	Growth of new blood vessels
PDGF	Migration and proliferation of fibroblasts and smooth muscle cells
FGF	Growth of new blood vessels
	Endothelial cell migration in damaged tissues
	Skeletal muscle development
TGF-β (beta)	Stimulates fibroblast chemotaxis
	Enhances collagen production
	Strong anti-inflammatory effect

VEGF vascular endothelial growth factor, *PDGF* platelet derived growth factor, *FGF* fibroblast growth factor, *TGF* transforming growth factor in sensitivity regarding follow-up of healing injuries due to increased resolution. Repeat imaging can be used to evaluate severity and the time course of injury. MRI can be used to determine prognosis by measuring the longitudinal length of muscle injury, which correlates to time lost from injury [9]. Severity of injury is determined by the severity of intramuscular edema, hemorrhage, and fiber injury, which in turn will also affect prognosis [8]. Ultrasound may be more favorable than MRI when cost and convenience are taken into account. Thus, ultrasound may be preferable if repeat examinations are planned to evaluate the ongoing healing process. Observation of remaining fluid collection may serve as an additional prognostic determinate in overall healing [10] (Fig. 9.2).

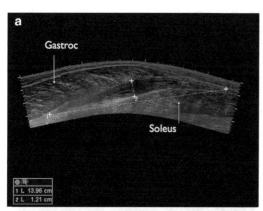

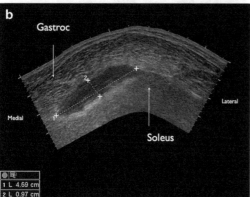

Fig. 9.2 **a** Ultrasound image, sagittal orientation. Hematoma in tissue plane dissecting *gastroc* muscle from the *soleus* muscle. **b** Ultrasound image, axial orientation. Hematoma in tissue plane dissecting *gastroc* muscle from the *soleus* muscle

For many patients, full recovery from muscle injury in the posterior leg may take up to several months before returning to previous pain-free activity level [10]. However, the sub-acute phase of injury begins long before then, and treatment choices can affect the extent and timing of recovery. Treatments aimed at the sub-acute phase are discussed at the end of the chapter and detailed in other chapters in this book.

Soleus

The soleus muscle is positioned deep to the gastroc. In considering primary muscle injuries it is largely ignored because until recently the soleus was thought rarely to get injured [11]. Several factors contribute to neglecting this muscle. Clinically an injury to the gastroc garnishes all the attention due to the dramatic presentation and frequency of occurrence, while a concomitant or isolated soleus injury is subtle and often goes unnoticed. Imaging studies may also underreport soleus injuries. Ultrasonography, although an excellent diagnostic tool, is very operator dependent, and an inexperienced examiner without a high index of suspicion may overlook an injury to the soleus. In addition, the deeper location of the soleus makes evaluation with ultrasound more difficult. Finally, the soleus is made up of predominately Type I (slow-twitch) fibers, a muscle type not typically associated with muscle strains. Consequently, soleus strain is thought unlikely and not commonly considered when patients have posterior leg pain. Despite these reasons for neglecting the soleus, it is an important injury to consider in the patient with sub-acute or chronic posterior leg pain, particularly if provoked by repetitive activity.

Injuries to the soleus can occur in various locations throughout the muscle. The two areas most affected are the musculotendinous junction and the myofascial junction. Musculotendinous junction strains are more common and occur at the distal intramuscular tendon or the proximal medial and lateral aponeuroses. The locations of the medial and lateral aponeuroses are just distal to the muscle origin, on the posterior tibia and fibula, respectively. The two pennate structures merge centrally to form the intramuscular central tendon as they move distally toward the Achilles tendon. Strains occurring away from the tendons are considered myofascial. Primarily, this occurs at the myofascial junction with the gastrocnemius or at the junction of the posterior compartment of the leg [11] (Fig. 9.3).

History and physical exam help to differentiate a soleus injury from a gastrocnemius injury. Soleus injury occurs during low-impact activity such as walking or jogging. Frequently, a sentinel event is lacking. Typical presentation symptoms include: calf tightness, stiffness, and worsening pain over the course of several days [7]. Palpation of the various aponeuroses, along with flexing the knee during examination, may help illicit

more objective findings. Knee flexion eliminates the confounding influence of the gastroc. If deemed clinically necessary, imaging with ultrasound or MRI can clarify diagnostic uncertainty. Due to the deeper location of the soleus, MRI is considered superior to ultrasound for determining degree of injury [11].

There is a paucity of literature regarding the treatment of soleus injury. This is likely due to the decreased frequency of soleus injury relative to gastrocnemius injuries and the challenges in diagnosing soleus injuries. This injury may also be underappreciated in current clinical practice because symptoms can often resemble that of delayed-onset muscle soreness [11]. However, these injuries should benefit from a similar

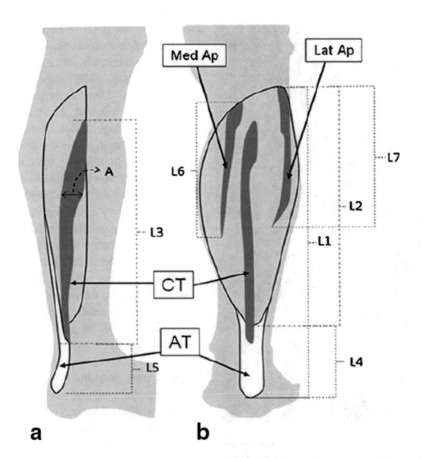

Fig. 9.3 a Sagittal view facing medial aspect of calf. **b** Posterior coronal view. *CT* Central tendon, *AT* Achilles tendon, *Med Ap* Medial aponeurosis, *Lat Ap* Lateral apo-

neurosis (Common location of plantaris strain in *bold*). (From [11]. Reprinted with permission from Springer Science+Business Media) treatment approach used for gastrocnemius injury described below.

Plantaris

The plantaris is an accessory muscle working in conjunction with the soleus and gastrocnemius muscles to provide a minimal amount of plantar flexion of the calf. The muscle belly itself is small, while the tendon is one of the largest in the body [12]. The plantaris muscle is absent in 7–10 % of the population [13, 14]. The plantaris muscle originates on the superior posterior aspect of the lateral femoral condyle, just medial to the lateral head of the gastrocnemius. The muscle belly of the plantaris travels from this origin, in an inferior obliquely medial direction extending an average 10 cm. The muscle belly then gives way to a long slender tendon whose course extends between the medial head of the gastrocnemius and soleus eventually accompanying the Achilles tendon to insert on the medial aspect of the calcaneus.

Injuries to the plantaris are often overlooked. Historically, prior to soft tissue imaging techniques such as MRI or ultrasound, surgical exploration was necessary to prove plantaris tendon rupture. Since imaging is not commonly performed in posterior leg muscle injuries, the true incidence of plantaris rupture is unknown. Further impairing incidence data, clinical suspicion of plantaris muscle injury can be delayed because strains of the muscle may lack a sentinel traumatic event. Plantaris injuries can occur in isolation or as a component of multiple tissue traumas accompanying an anterior cruciate ligament (ACL) tear, lateral compartment bone contusion, or arcuate ligament injury [14].

The evaluation of plantaris injuries begins with a thorough history. The clinician may need to assist the patient to recall symptom onset, acute or insidious, mechanism of injury and early clinical symptoms. Like gastrocnemius injuries, the mechanism usually combines forcibly extending the knee on a fixed dorsiflexed ankle. This history can understandably lead to misdiagnosis of plantaris injury as a strain to the medial head of the gastrocnemius [15]. This may be exacerbated by patient history that includes an inciting event with audible "pop" sensation. The clinician may expect the history to include pain; however, Allard describes two patients whose primary complaint consisted of vague muscle soreness and a cramping sensation [16]. Likewise, in the right clinical setting a differential diagnosis must also consider DVT.

Physical examination for a suspected plantaris rupture is frustratingly nonspecific. Pertinent physical findings consist of swelling in the posterior medial upper calf. This is in distinction to the medial head gastroc tear that usually occurs at the myotendinous junction. A tender, palpable mass can sometimes be appreciated just below the popliteal fossa. Visible hemorrhage may or may not be present. Full range of motion at the ankle and knee are possible. A false positive Homans' sign for DVT is also possible [16].

Imaging is not usually necessary or indicated to confirm a plantaris muscle or tendon tear. However, imaging is indicated for diagnostic clarification when DVT or neoplasm is considered. Characteristics of plantaris tear on MRI include a fluid presence interspersed between the gastroc and soleus [16]. This is in distinction to intramuscular edema seen with gastroc or soleus muscle strain. Although a concomitant gastroc strain is possible, an isointense gastroc and soleus muscles is typical, thereby assisting to differentiate this mass from neoplasm. A retracted muscle belly is seen with complete ruptures at the myotendinous junction.

MRI or ultrasonography is the modality of choice for imaging. The plantaris tendon is an avascular structure, so imaging displays an isointense mass between the gastrocnemius and soleus muscles [14, 16].

Ultrasonography provides a less costly alternative to MRI for assessment of plantaris injuries. Advancements in ultrasound have led to greatly improved resolution. Interpretation and assessment is operator dependent. Fluid collections between the gastroc and soleus are easily appreciated by ultrasound. Ultrasonography also offers the opportunity to simultaneously assess the leg for DVT.

Table 9.2 Comparison of posterior lower limb muscular injuries

	Plantaris tendon tear	Soleus injury	Gastrocnemius strain
History	Acute popping (+/−)	Ache	Explosive activity
	Insidious soreness, swelling, cramping	Worsening pain over days	Progressive swelling, pain
		Calf tightness, stiffness	
Physical	Associated knee pathology	Medial, lateral, or distal calf pain	Medial calf tenderness
Imaging	US or MRI	MRI preferred, US	US or MRI

US ultrasound, *MRI* magnetic resonance imaging

Treatment for plantaris injury is conservative. Management will be similar to gastrocnemius strain, often because the clinician is not initially thinking of possible injury to the plantaris muscle. Rest, ice, and nonsteroidal anti-inflammatory drugs (NSAIDs) are the modalities recommended. There has not been documented treatment with other therapeutic measures; however, those listed below may have benefits. Surgery is not necessary for confirmation of injury or treatment [16]. Although, surgery performed for diagnostic clarification has been done [15] (Table 9.2).

Severe/Prolonged or Delayed Recovery of Muscle Injuries in the Posterior Leg

Resolution of injuries to the posterior lower leg musculature depends on several factors. Most notably, the severity of muscle strain may dictate a prolonged course toward recovery. Strains are typically graded I–III to outline severity. Grade I strains involve partial muscle tears with no identifiable loss of muscle integrity. Grade II strains involve anywhere from 10 to 50% muscle disruption, while grade III muscle strains involve at least 50% loss of muscle integrity [17]. These more severe injuries in turn require a prolonged rehabilitative process and healing time. A variety of factors (premature return to play, poor treatment protocol, and delay in injury detection) may prolong healing and result in maladaptive restoration and chronic injury. This in turn increases scar tissue formation and tissue disorganization altering muscle function. Consequently, the muscle becomes dysfunctional and a source of chronic pain.

In severe strains, patients may require a period of non-weight bearing and immobilization until the muscle heals enough to tolerate ambulation. However, injuries that have reached the chronic phase are usually unresponsive to rest and will exhibit pain and weakness that limit function on resumption of activity. Therefore, treatments emphasizing restoration of structure and function are generally recommended for chronic strains. Eccentric exercises may be beneficial as they promote strengthening of passive tissue elements and have proven useful in chronic muscle tendinopathy [18]. Other treatments such as platelet-rich plasma (PRP) may provide chemokines and growth factors at a cellular level to create a local milieu to promote healing. Proprioceptive exercises along with biomechanical correction may help reduce symptoms and prevent or delay injury recurrence. Soft tissue mobilization and manual therapy techniques may reduce tissue adhesions, improve tissue organization, and stimulate a local healing response [19, 20].

Calcific Gastrocnemius Tendonitis

Calcific tendonitis has been observed as a cause of chronic posterior leg pain in few case reports dating back as early as 1981. This condition is primarily observed in the elderly. While calcium pyrophosphate dihydrate (CPPD) crystals are a relatively common finding in the gastrocnemius (incidence as high as 32% in patients with average age of 72), associated tendonitis is a rare cause of chronic pain [21]. In the case reports, the condition affected elderly women and symptoms included posterior knee pain with decreased knee flexion. Initial workup included plain radiographs followed by computed tomography (CT) and/or MRI. Patients responded to treatments including repeated local corticosteroid injection or surgical decompression after failed conservative management [21]. Newer minimally invasive techniques such as ultrasound-guided tenotomy may prove beneficial but as yet are unsubstantiated in the literature.

Chronic Exertional Compartment Syndrome

The lower extremity is comprised of four compartments including the anterior, lateral, superficial posterior, and deep posterior compartments. The gastrocnemius, soleus, and sural nerve make up the superficial posterior compartment. The deep posterior is made up of the flexor hallucis longus, flexor digitorum, tibialis posterior, posterior tibial nerve, and posterior tibial artery and vein. The deep posterior compartment is the most common cause of posterior compartment syndrome making up 45 % of all chronic exertional compartment syndrome (CECS) in the posterior lower extremity [22]. CECS occurs when increasing physical activity results in elevated intra-compartment pressures causing reduced regional blood flow to affected muscles. Poor flow in turn causes symptoms of ischemia, which include pain, paresthesias, cramping, and weakness. This condition is commonly seen in athletes (especially runners) under the age of 30 years affecting both males and females equally.

Diagnosis of CECS is made after thorough history and physical exam along with confirmatory testing. Complaints typically consist of recurrent reproducible pain with sustained exercise. This is the threshold at which blood flow becomes compromised due to muscle expansion during activity. After adequate rest the symptoms typically resolve. Confirmatory testing can be done by measuring intracompartmental pressure. Objective measures of CECS include a 1-min postexercise pressure greater than or equal to 30 mmHg and a 5-min postexercise pressure greater than or equal to 20 mmHg [23]. Other diagnostic techniques are investigational and include use of MRI or near-infrared spectroscopy (NIRS) [24]. Postexercise MRI may show increased signal on T2 images. NIRS measures oxygen saturation of hemoglobin in deep tissues

to demonstrate relative change in blood flow during activity versus rest [24].

Management of CECS includes both nonsurgical and surgical approaches. More conservative measures include activity cessation, reduction, or modification of gait, NSAIDs, stretching, or alternative activities. If there is no improvement after 6–12 weeks, surgical intervention should be considered. Surgical methods include subcutaneous fasciotomy. While surgery is more invasive, it remains the mainstay for long-term benefits. Risks of surgery include infection, hematoma, DVT, or peripheral nerve injury. Details of surgical evaluation and management can be found in Chap. 10.

Sural Nerve Entrapment

The sural nerve is a collateral branch of the tibial nerve which provides sensory function to the posterior lower leg. It traverses between the two heads of the gastrocnemius muscle before coursing through a fibrous arcade to the distal superficial lateral leg [25]. Entrapment of the sural nerve can result in chronic calf pain which is exacerbated by increasing physical activity [25]. Often symptoms can be confused with musculotendinous injury or vascular problems resulting in a delay in appropriate diagnosis and treatment.

The epidemiologic make up of people at risk for this condition include males between the ages of 30 and 60 years. Other risk factors include running and racquet sports; however, the condition has been seen in less-dangerous sports such as cycling and roller skating as well. The patient will report a history of chronic pain in the posterior aspect of the leg with exacerbation during activity. The pain may also radiate proximally or distally with exacerbation. Tenderness to palpation may be noted distal to the fibrous arcade in the area of the myotendinous junction of the Achilles tendon. Electrodiagnostic testing may aid diagnosis.

Treatment considerations include both operative and nonoperative therapy. Nonoperative measures which may include NSAIDs, therapeutic massage, and a stretching regimen have not demonstrated significant long-term benefits. Surgical intervention includes neurolysis and resection of the fibrous arcade. This may result in return to previous activity around 8 weeks with moderate pain relief [25].

Chronic Conditions (Table 9.3)

Therapeutic Options

Common therapeutic options available for patients presenting with sub-acute and chronic posterior leg strains include medications, manual therapies, and physical therapy modalities. These approaches are designed to reduce pain, improve function, hasten recovery, and reduce the chance of recurrence. A detailed discussion of specific rehabilitation strategies can be found in Chap. 11. Although common treatment strategies for posterior leg strains are discussed below, the interested reader is referred to Chap. 13 for additional information on complementary medical treatments.

Medications are used to treat pain and inflammation during the acute phase of injury; however, they are also used through the early stages of subacute injury for added pain reduction. The mechanism of action involves nonselective cyclooxygenase inhibition. This, in turn, prevents the formation of prostaglandins from arachidonic acid

[26–28]. NSAIDs have been studied and shown to decrease pain without having any adverse effect on recovery in terms of muscle fiber strength [28, 29]. While there have been many studies involving NSAID use, there is still discrepancy about the benefits and adverse effects when used as a treatment for soft tissue injury such as muscle strain. In the short term, NSAIDs have provided analgesia and improvements in muscle healing and function. However, in the long term, they have shown no benefits or even detrimental effects to the healing process [27, 30]. It is important to exercise caution or avoid NSAIDs use in patients who have a history of gastritis, gastroesophageal reflux disease (GERD), or intestinal ulcers.

Another important consideration when evaluating use of NSAIDs includes dosage of the medication. Over-the-counter NSAID doses provide analgesic and antipyretic effects. In order to achieve anti-inflammatory effects, the dose generally needs to be doubled [30]. Overall, NSAIDs should not be recommended in sub-acute and chronic injuries as they provide little benefit outside of the acute inflammatory phase. A better alternative in order to continue treating pain is acetaminophen. This medication has comparable analgesic efficacy to NSAIDs without the adverse effects associated with NSAID use [28].

Empirical use of corticosteroids is also a treatment for muscle strains. The risks and benefits of

Table 9.3 Differential diagnosis for chronic posterior leg pain

Diagnosis	Key features	Imaging studies
Medial tibial stress syndrome	Pain over posteromedial tibia	MRI, bone scan
Popliteal artery entrapment	Young men (<40 y/o), intermittent claudication	Arteriogram
Sural nerve entrapment	Paresthesia, sensory changes worse with activity	EMG
Deep vein thrombosis	Pain after prolonged period of immobility, recent travel	Duplex ultrasound
Chronic exertional compartment syndrome	Recurrent, reproducible pain after period of activity, young males and females (<30 y/o)	Compartment pressure testing, MRI, NIRS
Nerve root impingement	Radicular signs or symptoms, lower back pain	MRI
Chronic muscle strain	Continued pain or disability following injury	Ultrasound

y/o years old, *MRI* magnetic resonance imaging, *NIRS* near-infrared spectroscopy, *EMG* electromyography corticosteroid medications for sub-acute muscle strains is the topic of considerable debate. Corticosteroids are most commonly used to treat muscle injury by injecting the medication directly into the primary injury site. The patient should be apprised of the risks of such injections and the minimal amount of literature evidence of benefit to support the risk. Since a primary mechanism of action includes collagen inhibition, there is at least a theoretical risk of tendon rupture. This risk has not been studied in large-scale randomized controlled trials. Case studies are the best evidence for this risk [31, 32]. There are numerous variables that may contribute to a postinjection tendon failure (i.e., incomplete recovery from the primary injury, rapid escalation to risky activities, age, and random tendon failure), thus, clearly identifying the contribution of corticosteroid injection to the tendon failure is challenging. Other less concerning adverse effects include subcutaneous fat necrosis and skin depigmentation. Typically, systemic adverse effects do not occur with injections [33]. However, repeated injections may have adverse systemic effects. This is due to a portion of the injected corticosteroid becoming systemically absorbed. This can lead to adrenal suppression and osteoblastic activity depression [31]. Anaphylaxis is also a theoretical concern but has not been well documented in literature [31].

The more common corticosteroids used for injection include triamcinolone and dexamethasone. This is, in part, due to their potency. When compared to hydrocortisone, triamcinolone has five times the anti-inflammatory activity, while dexamethasone has 25 times more anti-inflammatory activity [33]. Short-term use of local corticosteroid injection has demonstrated good results in sub-acute cases that have not responded well to initial conservative management [34]. To date, there have not been extensive studies which demonstrate the appropriate dose or treatment to maximize benefit without having deleterious effects (Table 9.4).

Medications can also be delivered in conjunction with therapeutic modality by phonophoresis and iontophoresis. Both interventions allow for medication to be topically administered directly

Table 9.4 Corticosteroid potency

Medication	Relative potency
Dexamethasone	25
Triamcinolone	5
Hydrocortisone	1

over the injured structure. In the case of phonophoresis, medication in gel form is transferred through use of the pulsatile waves of therapeutic ultrasound. Phonophoresis using gel-Dimethyl-sulfoxide (DMSO) has been shown to improve muscle healing when compared to pulsatile ultrasound alone or gel-DMSO administration alone [35]. The method is through decrease of pro-inflammatory cells [36]. A hypothesis for the mechanism of action for phonophoresis is that the mechanical stimulus provided by ultrasound wave results in activation of signal transduction pathways that are involved in muscle repair [35]. Medication is also administered topically through use of iontophoresis. This process takes advantage of the polarity of a medication, which is then electrically charged to allow penetration into the surface of the target muscle. Dexamethasone has commonly been used as the medication of choice for iontophoresis [37]. Some advantages of iontophoresis and phonophoresis include enhanced depth of penetration of medication, less pain, less risk of systemic effects, and skin remains intact, which helps lower risk of infection. Adverse effects are minimal and include tingling, skin irritation, and thermal injury [38]. A primary limitation of this technique is that the stratum corneum layer of the skin must be intact for effective penetration of medication [38].

More recently, treatment emphasis has been placed on providing growth factors to assist in muscle regeneration. Some of these growth factors include transforming growth factor (TGF-β1 [beta-1]) and FGF as well as multiple cytokines [39, 40]. These specific treatments are aimed directly at expediting the sub-acute phase of injury. The most common application of this method is known as PRP therapy. Other variations for this approach include application of platelet-rich fibrin, fibrin sealant, platelet concentrate, and platelet-rich fibrin matrix [41]. PRP originated in the surgical setting where it was used to promote postoperative tissue healing. While fibrin-like substances were first being used as early as 1970, it was not until 1987 that the term PRP came in to favor. The current theory behind PRP is that platelets contain several growth factors necessary in the regeneration process following injury. PRP is obtained from autologous blood then prepared using extracorporeal techniques to increase platelet concentration prior to being injected into the area of tissue damage [41]. In addition to increased speed of recovery, PRP is also thought to enhance the quality of tissue repair [42]. In animal studies, PRP has been shown to improve time of recovery for repetitive muscle injuries. However, there was no proven benefit with single lengthening (eccentric) contraction injury model [42]. In addition to animal studies, there have been several studies done on PRP in humans; however, the quality of evidence is limited due to preponderance of studies that were non-blinded and had no long-term follow-up [40]. While the concepts behind PRP are promising, significant questions remain regarding both the overall effectiveness and specific application of this treatment. This is, in part, due to the lack of standardization behind the method. Currently, there are no definitive protocols for the amount, consistency, or methods of PRP use [41]. To date, there have been no randomized trials that have studied PRP injections for the purposes of muscle healing [43]. While PRP appears promising, there is still potential for adverse effects. Although a theoretical concern regarding PRP includes a systemic increase in growth factors, which could lead to neoplastic outcomes, there is no current data to support this notion [40, 44]. There is also no data regarding long-term adverse effects.

It should be noted that at the elite level, a review of current guidelines regarding anti-doping should take place prior to PRP treatment. In 2010, the World Anti-Doping Agency (WADA) banned intramuscular PRP injections; however, intraarticular and intra- or peri-tendinous use was permitted if clearly documented [41]. Also, use of individual growth factors including insulin-like growth factor 1 (IGF-1), vascular endothelial growth factor (VEGF), and platelet-derived growth factor (PDGF) are specifically banned by WADA. The lack of uniformity regarding PRP products potentially increases the compliance risk for elite athletes and should be taken into account when considering use of this treatment option.

Therapeutic interventions that do not involve pharmacotherapy include Kinesio taping, compression sleeves/stockings, and heel lifts or other biomechanical correction. Kinesio taping is a therapeutic method involving a specific style of tape that has been used as a supplemental treatment for various musculoskeletal injuries. A proposed mechanism of Kinesio tape is related to the mechanical elevation of the skin from the underlying fascia. This process is thought to allow for increased blood flow, oxygenation, and lymphatic flow to the tissue. The end result is decreased inflammation and improved muscle function. This may facilitate improved healing and quicker return to activity following sub-acute injury. While this theory appears promising, there is little evidence to support these claims. The most recent research assessing oxygenation and increased blood flow did not demonstrate any benefit from Kinesio taping [45]. However, this study was only performed on healthy individuals. While there is limited evidence-based data to demonstrate its effectiveness, Kinesio taping continues to be widely used for musculoskeletal injuries.

Compression sleeves are thought to increase the muscle pump effect of the calf muscle. This, in turn, allows for increased blood flow and oxygenation to allow for better muscle function and improved healing potential [46]. Compression may also help decrease pain and swelling involved in acute muscle strain injuries [10]. In the sub-acute phase of healing, compression sleeves assist in early activity. During activity, compression sleeves increase tissue perfusion and oxygenation; however, the duration of this effect is unknown [47]. Compression sleeves are also used in chronic injuries to reduce the chance of recurrence and improve ease of activity.

Heel lifts are therapeutic devices that provide a mechanical change to normal gait. The lift acts as a support that increases plantar flexion and, in turn, shortens the length of the gastrocnemius muscle. This decreases tension on the gastrocnemius, which may facilitate pain modification and allow for a more timely recovery. One study demonstrated that heel lifts between 1.9 and 5.7 cm decreased gastrocnemius muscle activity in normal ground-level walking in men [48]. This benefit may be minimal in women who regularly wear high-heeled shoes [48]. There are no current recommendations on the adequate height of heel lifts or the duration for which a lift should be used. It should be noted that if a chronic heel lift is used it may predispose the patient to equinus type contractures and associated problems.

References

1. Anderson M, Hall S, Martin M. Sports injury management. 2nd ed. Philadelphia: Lippincott Williams and Wilkins; 2000. (Chapter 5, Tissue healing & wound care; p. 106–7).
2. Witte M, Barbul A. General principles of wound healing. Surg Clin North Am. 1997;77(3):509–28.
3. Kumar V, Abbas AK, Fausto N. Robbins and Cotran pathologic basis of disease. 7th ed. Philadelphia: Elsevier Saunders; 2005. (Chapter 3, Tissue renewal & repair: regeneration, healing, & fibrosis; p. 96–7).
4. Jarvinen TAH, Kaariainen M, Jarvinen M, Kalimo H. Muscle strain injuries. Curr Opin Rheumatol. 2000;12:155–61.
5. Cutlip R, Baker B, Hollander M. Injury and adaptive mechanisms in skeletal muscle. J Electromyogr Kinesiol. 2009;19:358–72.
6. Campbell RSD, Dunn AJ. Radiological interventions for soft tissue injuries in sport. Br J Radiol. 2012;85(1016):1186–93.
7. Dixon JB. Gastrocnemius vs. soleus strain: how to differentiate and deal with calf muscle injuries. Curr Rev Musculoskelet Med. 2009;2(2):74–7.
8. Douis H, Gillett M, James SL. Imaging in the diagnosis, prognostication, and management of lower limb muscle injury. Semin Musculoskelet Radiol. 2011;15(1):27–41.
9. Song H, Nakazato K, Nakajima H. Effect of increased excursion of the ankle on the severity of acute eccentric contraction-induced strain injury in the gastrocnemius. Am J Sports Med. 2004;32(5):1263–9.
10. Kwak H, Lee K, Han Y. Ruptures of the medial head of the gastrocnemius (severity of acute eccentric contraction-induced strain). Clin Imaging. 2006;30(1):48–53.
11. Balius R, Alomar X, Rodas G, Miguel-Perez M, Pedret C, Dobado MC, Koulouris G. The soleus muscle: MRI, anatomic and histologic findings in cadavers with clinical correlation of strain injury distribution. Skeletal Radiol. 2013;42(4):521–30.
12. Biel A. Trail guide to the body. 2nd edn. Boulder: Books of Discovery; 2001. (Chapter 7, Leg & Foot; p. 300).
13. Jones GB. Pathology of Ruptured Plantaris. Br Med J. 1945;1(4407):876.
14. Helms CA, Fritz RC, Garvin GJ. Plantaris muscle injury: evaluation with MR imaging. Radiology. 1995;195(1):201–3.
15. Hamilton W, Klostermeier T, Lim EV, Moulton JS. Surgically documented rupture of the plantaris muscle: a case report and literature review. Foot Ankle Int. 1997;18(8):522–3.
16. Allard J, Bancroft J, Porter G. Imaging of Plantaris muscle rupture. Clin Imaging. 1992;16(1):55–8.
17. Saxena A, St. Louis M, Fournier M. Vibration and pressure wave therapy for calf strains: a proposed treatment. Muscles Ligaments Tendons J. 2013;3(2):60–2.
18. LaStayo PC, Woolf JM, Lewek MD, et al. Eccentric muscle contractions: their contribution to injury, prevention, rehabilitation, and sport. J Orthop Sports Phys Ther. 2003;33:557–71.
19. Looney B, Srokose T, Fernandez-de-las-Penas C, et al. Graston instrument soft tissue mobilization and home stretching for management of plantar heel pain: a case series. J Manipulative Physiol Ther. 2011;34(2):138–42.
20. Miners AL, Bougie TL. Chronic Achilles tendinopathy: a case study of treatment incorporating active and passive tissue warm-up, Graston Technique, ART, eccentric exercise, and cryotherapy. J Can Chiropr Assoc. 2011;55(4):269–78.
21. Iguchi Y, Ihara N, Hijioka A, Uchida S, et al. Calcifying tendonitis of the gastrocnemius. JBJS(B). 2002;84B(3):431–2.
22. George CA, Hutchinson MR. Chronic exertional compartment syndrome. Clin J Sports Med. 2012;31:307–19.
23. Pedowitz RA, Hargens AR, Mubarak SJ, et al. Modified criteria for the objective diagnosis of chronic compartment syndrome of the leg. Am J Sports Med. 1990;18(1):35–40.
24. Dunn JC, Waterman BR. Chronic exertional compartment syndrome of the leg in the military. Clin J Sports Med. 2014;33:693–705.
25. Fabre T, Montero C, Gaujard E, et al. Chronic calf pain in athletes due to sural nerve entrapment. Am J Sports Med. 2000;28(5):679–82.
26. Dahners LE, Mullis BH. Effects of nonsteroidal anti-inflammatory drugs on bone formation and soft-tissue healing. J Am Acad Orthop Surg. 2004;12(3):139–43.
27. Almekinders LC. Anti-inflammatory treatment of muscular injuries in sport: an update of recent studies. Sports Med. 1999;28(6):383–88.
28. Paoloni JA, Orachard JW. The use of therapeutic medications for soft-tissue injuries in sports medicine. Med J Aust. 2005;183(7):384–88.
29. Obremsky W, Seaber A, Ribbeck B, Garrett W. Biomechanical and histologic assessment of a controlled muscle strain injury treated with piroxicam. Am J Sports Med. 1994;22(4):558–61.

30. Hertel J. The role of nonsteroidal anti-inflammatory drugs in the treatment of acute soft tissue injuries. J Athl Train. 1997;32(4):350–8.

31. Fredberg U. Local corticosteroid injection in sport: review of literature and guidelines for treatment. Scand J Med Sci Sports. 1997;7(3):131–9.

32. Nichols AW. Complications associated with the use of corticosteroids in the treatment of athletic injuries. Clin J Sport Med. 2005;15(5):370–75.

33. Buckwalter JA. Drug treatment of soft tissue injuries efficacy and tissue effects. Iowa Orthop J. 1993;13:40–8.

34. Paavola M, Kannus P, Jarvinen TA, Jarvinen TL, Jozsa L, Jarvinen M. Treatment of tendon disorders. Is there a role for corticosteroid injection? Foot Ankle Clin. 2002;7(3):501–13.

35. Silveira PCL, da Silva LA, Tromm C, Scheffer D, de Souza CT, Ricardo AP. Effects of therapeutic pulsed ultrasound and dimethylsulfoxide phonophoresis on oxidative stress parameters after injury induced by eccentric exercise. Ultrasonics. 2012;52(5):650–4.

36. Engelmann J, Vitto MF, Cesconetto PA, Silveira PCL, Possato JC, Pinho RA, Paula MM, Victor EG, De Souza CT. Pulsed ultrasound and dimethylsulfoxide gel treatment reduces the expression of pro-inflammatory molecules in an animal model of muscle injury. Ultrasound Med Biol. 2012;38(8):1470–5.

37. Gurney AB, Wascher DC. Absorption of dexamethasone sodium phosphate in human connective tissue using iontophoresis. Am J Sports Med. 2008;36(4):753–9.

38. Kassan DG, Lynch AM, Siller MJ. Physical enhancement of dermatologic drug delivery: Iontophoresis and phonophoresis. J Am Acad Dermatol. 1996;34(4):657–66.

39. Mishra A, Woodall J, Vieira A. Treatment of tendon and muscle using platelet-rich plasma. Clin Sports Med. 2009;28(1):113–25.

40. Hamilton B, Best TM. Platelet-enriched plasma and muscle strain injuries: challenges imposed by the burden of proof. Clin J Sport Med. 2011;21(1):31–6.

41. Engebretsen L, Steffen K, Alsousou J, Anitua E, Bachl N, Devilee R, Everts P, Hamilton B, Huard J, Jenoure P, Kelberine F, Kon E, Maffulli N, Matheson G, Mei-Dan O, Menetrey J, Phillipon M, Randelli P, Schamasch P, Schwellnus M, Vernec A, Verrall G. IOC consensus paper on the use of platelet-rich plasma in sports medicine. Br J Sports Med. 2010;44(15):1072–81.

42. Harmon KG. Muscle injuries and PRP: what does the science say? Br J Sports Med. 2010;44(9):616–7.

43. Andia I, Sanchez M, Maffulli N. Platelet rich plasma therapies for sports muscle injuries: any evidence behind clinical practice? Expert Opin Biol Ther. 2011;11(4):509–18.

44. Foster TE, Puskas BL, Mandelbaum BR, Gerhardt MB, Rodeo SA. Platelet-rich plasma: from basic science to clinical applications. Am J Sports Med. 2009;37(11):2259–72.

45. Stedge HL, Kroskie RM, Docherty CL. Kinesio taping and the circulation and endurance ratio of the gastrocnemius muscle. J Athl Train. 2012;47(6):635–42.

46. Perrey S. Compression garments: evidence for their physiological effects. The engineering of sport 7. Vol. 2. Paris: Springer-Verlag; 2008. (Chapter 40; p. 319–28).

47. Coza A, Dunn J, Anderson B, Nigg B. Effects of compression on muscle tissue oxygenation at the onset of exercise. J Strength Cond Res. 2012;26(6):1631–7.

48. Lee KH, Matteliano A, Medige J, Smiehorowski T. Electromyographic changes of leg muscles with heel lift: therapeutic implications. Arch Phys Med Rehabil. 1987;68(5 Pt 1):298–301.

Surgical Treatment of Posterior Leg Injuries

10

Zachary C. Leonard

Introduction

Muscular injuries to the posterior leg are fairly common. These injuries are often subtle and require a thorough history and physical exam to properly diagnose. Acute injuries to the Achilles tendon can present in a similar fashion and are often the focus of clinical concern during the evaluation of posterior leg injuries. As such, many muscular injuries are often misdiagnosed as an Achilles tendon injury. The examiner must keep a high index of suspicion to delineate muscular injuries from Achilles tendon injury. Prior to deciding which injuries will require surgical intervention, the examiner must completely evaluate the injury and the resulting loss of function. The evaluation begins with a complete history, which includes age, past medical history including medications, previous injuries, and most importantly mechanism of injury.

Mechanism of injury is crucial, as the examiner can understand the position of the limb and direction of force, thus localizing which muscles would be at risk of injury. Understanding whether the injury was a noncontact, contact, or crush-style mechanism along with knowing the amount of energy (high or low) can help determine severity, the risk for complications, and subsequent treatment. Timing of injury and presentation is also critical. Many of these injuries can initially look benign, but progressive inflammation and swelling can lead to acute compartment syndrome.

Physical exam is fundamental in the diagnosis of these injuries and requires a thorough understanding of the anatomy (Fig. 10.1). A good physical examination begins with inspection. The examiner should look at the limb evaluating the skin for any compromise as well as swelling, bruising, redness, or deformity. Palpation of the limb aids in further localizing the area of injury as well as evaluating the fullness of the compartment. Thoroughly strength testing each musculotendinous unit in the injured area will facilitate isolation of the affected muscle.

Radiography is rarely helpful in the diagnosis of muscular injuries but can rule out concomitant fractures, deformity, and complications such as myositis ossificans. Advanced imaging, however, can provide valuable information in the diagnosis of muscular injuries. Ultrasound can be used to confirm muscular strains or ruptures, but is operator dependent. Magnetic resonant imaging (MRI) can be a useful adjunct to the history and exam, especially if the diagnosis is in question or surgical intervention is being contemplated. MRI gives detailed anatomical information that can confirm the injury and help with preoperative planning. For example, the amount of retraction present in cases of muscle ruptures can be measured on MRI. Fascial defects can also be localized on MRI.

Z. C. Leonard (✉)
Orthopedic Surgery, Advanced Center for Orthopedics,
Marquette, MI, USA
e-mail: zcleonard@gmail.com

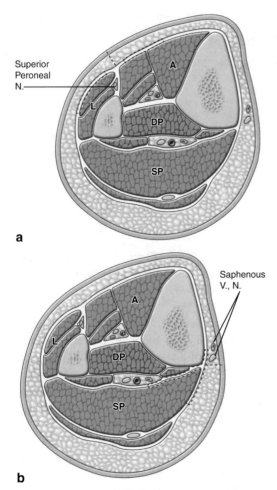

a

b

Fig. 10.1 Compartment illustration. These cross sections at mid-calf level show the four compartments of the leg and their contents. Specifically, the superficial posterior *(SP)* and deep posterior *(DP)* compartments. The SP compartment contains the gastrocnemius, plantaris, soleus, and sural nerve. The DP contains the posterior tibial, flexor halluces longus, flexor digitorum longus musculotendinous units along with the tibial nerve, posterior tibial artery and vein

After a complete history and physical exam has been obtained and the muscular injury has been defined with or without the addition of advanced imaging, the examiner must go through a systematic process to determine optimal treatment. First and foremost, the examiner must stratify the patient's risk of compartment syndrome. If acute compartment syndrome is identified, immediate surgical intervention is warranted. It is important to remember that although a patient's

exam can initially be benign, compartment syndrome can develop hours or days after an injury and patients should be appropriately counseled about this risk [1]. The specifics of compartment syndrome evaluation and treatment are detailed later in this chapter.

In the absence of acute compartment syndrome, most posterior leg muscle injuries can be treated conservatively. Occasionally, surgical intervention is indicated. This determination must be tailored on a patient-by-patient basis. Pertinent considerations include the type of injury, level of disability and loss of function from the injury, patient's age and activity level, and any other medical comorbidity that could affect outcome.

Gastrocnemius Injury

Gastrocnemius injuries are the most common of all posterior leg injuries. A strain of the medial head of the gastrocnemius is referred to as "tennis leg." In addition, the gastrocnemius is the most superficial therefore most likely to sustain a contact injury resulting in a muscle contusion. Contracture of the gastrocnemius is fairly common in the general population further putting this muscle at risk of strain or rupture.

Conservative treatment is the mainstay of gastrocnemius muscular injuries. Rarely, a complete rupture at the musculotendinous junction may require surgical repair. This would be diagnosed by marked weakness on plantar flexion with a bulge over the proximal muscle belly from retraction, similar to the commonly observed "Popeye" deformity resulting from proximal retraction of the biceps brachii muscle. Operative indications would include complete muscle rupture with inability to plantarflex through the ankle or a large partial tear resulting in intolerable weakness to the patient.

Surgical repair of a ruptured gastrocnemius can be approached in two patient positions: prone or lateral on a beanbag with operative side down. This is surgeon preference; however, each approach has its advantages. The prone position allows a direct posterior approach that can be extended to allow full visualization of the proximal and distal ends of the rupture. It also allows inline traction to be placed on the proximal end of the rupture to regain length if retraction did not allow direct tension free repair. Disadvantage of the posterior approach is a directly posterior positioned scar can be symptomatic to the patient. Also, the sural nerve can be injured during a posterior approach as it often crosses the operative field. The surgeon must identify and protect this neurovascular structure. Additionally, in very rare circumstances, the prone position can lead to blindness due to an increase in intra-orbital pressure. Although this risk is typically associated with extensive spine surgery, it is a devastating complication and should be a consideration during surgical planning. The lateral position with the operative side down allows a more minimally invasive technique to be used with a medial positioned incision. This type of incision allows the surgeon to more easily identify and protect the sural nerve reducing the risk of nerve injury. This positioning also avoids the risk of blindness. Another advantage of the lateral position is placement of a scar on the medial side of the calf is often more cosmetically appealing and less bothersome for the patient.

Regardless of the approach used, the elements of the surgery remain the same. First, a skin incision is made longitudinally of adequate length to have access to the proximal and distal ends of the rupture. Often, a 5–8 cm incision is suitable for this purpose. The dissection continues through the subcutaneous fat tissue being careful to coagulate any crossing venous bleeders to prevent postoperative hematoma formation. Next, the crural fascia is incised in line with the skin incision. This exposes the superficial posterior compartment. The most superficial structure is the gastrocnemius. In the setting of a recent injury, a hematoma will be noted upon entering the superficial posterior compartment. Once the tear is identified, the hematoma and any interposed fibrous tissue must be debrided, so that direct apposition of viable muscle can take place. Depending on the strength of the tissue, #2 or 2.0 fiberwire suture may be used to sew the ruptured ends to each other. A locking suture stitch technique

(Krackow or Kessler stitch) will strengthen purchase in muscle tissue and help prevent pull through (Fig. 10.2). Additionally, the ankle may need to be placed into plantar flexion, relaxing the gastrocnemius, thus taking tension off of the repair. Knee flexion can also aid reducing tension on the repair as the gastrocnemius origin is on the femur. The patient should also be given muscle relaxation from the anesthesia team. The surgeon should be aware of the tension of the repair as well as the position of the ankle and knee at the time of the repair, which becomes important in postoperative splinting and rehabilitation protocol. After an adequate repair has apposed the ruptured ends of the muscle, the surgical wound closure should be done in layers. The crural fascia should be repaired with an absorbable vicryl suture (usually 3-0) to prevent any postoperative muscle herniation through the defect. The skin should then be apposed in a tension-free manner; an absorbable monocryl suture can be used for a cosmetic closure that does not require suture removal.

After closure, a splint should be placed with the ankle in a position of tension-free plantar flexion as determined intraoperatively. The splint is usually only below the knee, however, it may be extended above the knee if needed for the repair to remain tension free. The splint remains in place for 2 weeks, and then it is removed for inspection of the incision and transition to partial weight bearing in a cam walker. Often, a heel lift is used to keep the ankle in equinus and reduce the tension on the repair. The height of the heel lift is determined by the surgeon, taking the amount of tension on the repair in mind. At 4–6 weeks post-op, gentle range of motion is begun under the guidance of a physical therapist. At 8–10 weeks, strengthening activities are advanced. Return to play is sports specific but usually occurs by 4–6 months.

Soleus Injury

Isolated soleus muscle ruptures appear to be uncommon and have been infrequently described in the literature. Indications for operative repair

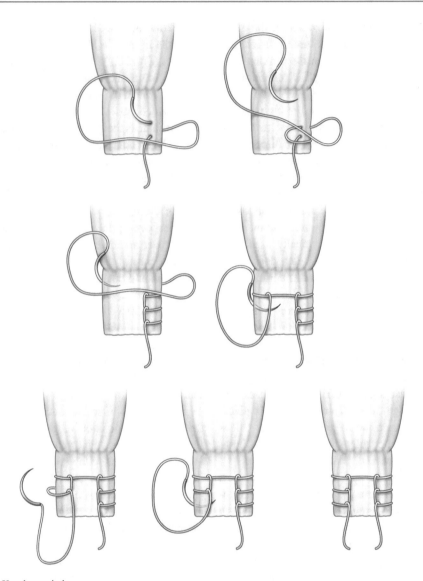

Fig. 10.2 Krackow stitch

would be rare but include marked weakness on plantar flexion and disability after appropriate conservative treatment. Rest, ice, compression, and elevation along with cam boot or short leg walking cast immobilization for comfort are the treatments of choice until the pain and disability dissipate. If symptoms persist, physical therapy should be employed to focus on range of motion and strengthening. If over 6 months to 1 year of disability persist after appropriate treatment, surgical treatment may be considered. Similar techniques as described above for gastrocnemius ruptures are used. Pertinent differences do exist,

however. The soleus muscle is the deep layer of the superficial posterior compartment of the leg. It lies underneath the gastrocnemius and originated on the posterior surface of the tibia, fibula, and interosseous membrane. It, therefore, does not cross the knee joint as the gastrocnemius does. It may be approached from a posterior or lateral approach. If approached posteriorly, the gastrocnemius tendon will need to be split to gain access to the soleus. Repair should be done in a similar fashion as described above for the gastrocnemius muscle. Patients' postoperative course should also be followed as above.

Plantaris Injury

The plantaris is often considered a vestigial muscle. It lies in the superficial posterior compartment of the leg and may have a limited role in augmenting plantar flexion at the ankle. Given its limited function, minimal long-term disability occurs when it is ruptured. This fact makes the plantaris a good donor tendon to augment local surgical repairs (most often the Achilles tendon). Treatment of plantaris injuries is conservative and should follow a similar approach as outline for soleus muscle injury.

Tibialis Posterior Injury

The tibialis posterior is the dynamic support to hold the height of the medial longitudinal arch. Lengthening of this musculotendinous unit can lead to pes planovalgus deformity (acquired flatfoot). Muscular tears or ruptures are infrequent as the majority of injury occurs more distally along the tendon near its insertion on the navicular. There are no reports in the literature of posterior tibialis rupture at the muscle level. All reported cases are tendon ruptures more distally. However, if a complete rupture did occur and weakness on plantar flexion and inversion through the ankle resulted, operative repair should be considered. A repair would not only improve residual weakness but would also prevent an acquired flatfoot deformity from forming due to loss of dynamic support of the posterior tibialis.

Surgical approach to the posterior tibialis can be done prone or in the lateral decubitus position with the operative side down allowing exposure to the medial aspect of the distal leg. Regardless of the position chosen, a posteromedial approach to the distal leg just proximal to the ankle should be employed. An 8–10 cm incision on the posterior medial crest of the tibia should be made. The crural fascia is split longitudinally and may be reflected posteriorly allowing entrance into the deep posterior compartment. Care should be taken not to dissect posterior to this region, as the neurovascular bundle lies just posterior to this area. Do not forget that posterior to the medial malleolus the order of structures from anterior to posterior goes tibialis posterior, flexor digitorum longus (FDL), tibial artery, nerve and vein, then the flexor hallucis longus (FHL; the mnemonic Tom, Dick, and, Harry helps in remembering the order of these structures). Once the muscle belly of the posterior tibialis is identified, the interposed hematoma and fibrous tissue should be debrided. Nonabsorbable suture such as #2 or 2-0 fiberwire can be used for the repair in a similar fashion as described for repair of the gastrocnemius. The split in the crural fascia should be repaired with an absorbable vicryl suture to prevent muscle herniation through the fascial defect. Skin closure should be done with a 3-0 nylon suture in simple or horizontal mattress configuration. A below knee splint should then be placed with the ankle in slight plantar flexion and inversion to take stress off the repair. At 2 weeks, the patient may be transitioned to partial weight bearing in a cam walker with the ankle maintained in slight plantar flexion and inversion. At 4–6 weeks, gentle range of motion exercises can be employed under physical therapy guidance. Strengthening may begin at 8–10 weeks, with return to sport at 4–6 months.

Flexor Digitorum Longus Injury

The FDL is responsible for flexion at the distal interphalangeal joint in the lesser toes. It has tendinous slip interconnections with the FHL in the plantar aspect of the foot. Additionally, the flexor hallucis brevis assists lesser-toe flexion at the proximal IP joint as well as the MTP joint. Therefore, ruptures of the FDL can be compensated for by the patient through FHL and flexor digitorum brevis (FDB) function and rarely leads to severe disability. There are no reports in the literature of isolated FDL rupture or results of FDL muscle repairs. Theoretically, if substantial weakness did result from a FDL muscle rupture, surgical repair could be considered. A similar approach to the repair of the posterior tibialis should be employed. Again, it is paramount not to injure the neurovascular bundle that sits directly posterior to the FDL in the retromalleolar region. Splinting and postoperative rehab should follow as described above for posterior tibialis repair.

Flexor Hallucis Longus Injury

The FHL is the main flexor of the big toe at the interphalangeal joint. This musculotendinous unit can be injured from a hyperdorsiflexion force. There are a couple of reports of injury at the musculotendinous region of the FHL. The majority of these injuries are treated conservatively, especially acutely. If an unacceptable loss of toe flexion or substantial weakness resulted after FHL muscle tear or rupture, then operative repair may be considered. Again, a prone position or lateral decubitus position with the operative side down would both be appropriate. A posterior medial approach through an 8–10 cm incision centered midway between the lateral malleolus and the Achilles tendon should be used. The crural fascia should be incised in line with the skin incision and the Achilles tendon should be retracted posteriorly and laterally. Once the deep posterior compartment is incised longitudinally, the muscle belly of the FHL can be identified. Again, dissection medial to the FHL should be avoided to prevent injury to the posterior neurovascular bundle. The interposed fibrous clot should be debrided and a nonabsorbable suture should be used for repair. The ankle and hallux may be flexed to help appose the proximal and distal ends of the rupture. Postoperative splinting should also be done in this position to limit tension on the repair. A similar postoperative course should be followed as for the tibialis posterior and FDL repairs described above.

Posterior Compartment Syndrome

Posterior compartment syndrome is a dreaded complication that can arise from any muscle injury to the posterior leg. The fascial compartments posteriorly (both superficial and deep) have a confined space and cannot tolerate substantial swelling. Increased pressure can lead to compression of the neurovascular structures as well as compression of the muscle leading to necrosis [2]. The diagnosis can either be made by clinically or quantitatively by doing compartment pressure testing. Clinical diagnosis is based on the physical exam taking into account the clinical picture. The classic "5 P's" of compartment syndrome should be evaluated. These include pain, pallor, paresthesias, paralysis, and pulselessness. On physical exam, swelling and firmness on palpation is noted. Pain with passive range of motion of the toes is often present. Also, pain out of proportion and pain not responsive to medications are worrisome signs of an impending compartment syndrome. Pallor, paresthesias, paralysis, and pulselessness are all late findings. If the physical exam is inconclusive, compartment pressure monitoring may be used to objectively decide treatment. In general, compartment pressures above 35 mmHg or within 30 mmHg of the diastolic blood pressure indicates compartment syndrome [1].

Once the diagnosis of acute compartment syndrome has been made, compartment fasciotomy becomes a surgical emergency. A compartment fasciotomy relieves compression on the muscle and neurovascular structures. As discussed above, the posterior leg is made of posterior and deep compartments. Fasciotomy of both compartments is recommended if a posterior compartment syndrome is present. Patient positioning is not critical, as fasciotomy may be done in supine, lateral, or prone positions. An open approach is the gold standard treatment. An arthroscopic assisted technique can also be used to allow a more minimally invasive approach. With this, smaller incisions can be used. It should be noted regardless of the approach, the same neurovascular structures must be avoided. For a standard open approach, posterior medially based incision allows easy release of the compartments. Typically an 8–10 cm longitudinal incision just posterior to the posterior diaphysis of the tibia is made centered 10 cm proximal to the medial malleolus. The saphenous nerve and vein are at risk and should be identified and bluntly retracted in the superficial layer. The crural fascia is then identified and splint longitudinally. Blunt release of the crural fascia should be done proximally and distally as far as possible allowing complete release of the superficial compartment and to prevent postoperative muscle herniation through a small fascial defect. The posterior tibial tendon and muscle is identified and retracted bluntly posteriorly. This allows visualization of the deep posterior compartment fascia. This deep compartment fascia is split longitudinally both proximally and distally exposing the deep posterior compartment musculature. The muscle most easily visualized will be the FDL on the posterior aspect of the tibial. At this point, the compartments are completely decompressed. For documentation purposes, compartment pressure testing may be done again at this point. A thorough evaluation should be done of the compartments. Viability of the muscle can be determined by color, consistency, contractibility, and capacity to bleed. Any non-viable tissue should be debrided [3]. Nonviable tissue often takes on a grayish hue, becomes easily friable, loses its ability to contract, and does not bleed. If the viability of the tissue is uncertain, leave it and reevaluate on repeat washout in 48–72 h to allow the tissue to demarcate [4, 5].

At this point, the entire wound should be copiously irrigated to clean it of any contaminates. The fasciotomy should be left open so the compartments remain decompressed. The only closure required is skin. Vicryl suture can be used to close the subcutaneous and fat layer of skin. Staples or nylon suture should then be used to close the skin. If the tension on the tissues does not allow a tension-free closure, a wound vac may be employed. Often after the wound vac is in place for 48–72 h, the skin may be closed. However, if closure is still not possible, definitive closure with skin grafting should be done within 10 days to 2 weeks.

The most important component of compartment syndrome is early detection and treatment. The physician must keep a high index of suspicion and repeat examinations are critical. If caught early, the detrimental effects of this serious complication can be averted.

Chronic Compartment Syndrome

The term chronic compartment syndrome includes two separate entities: chronic exertional compartment syndrome and missed compartment syndrome with residual effects . The latter of the

two is discussed below in post-injury equinus contractures. This section will focus on chronic exertional compartment syndrome. This term describes a temporary activity-related increase in compartment pressure causing ischemic pain and sometimes damage to the tissues. This pain is often recurrent and associated with repetitive activity. Usually, the pain subsides with rest and often with no permanent sequela on the tissues. Again, compartment pressure testing is utilized to confirm diagnosis. A resting compartment pressure of > 15 and/or > 30 mmHg at 1 min postexercise and/or > 20 mmHg at 5 min postexercise are the conventional parameters for diagnosis [6, 7].

Once the diagnosis has been made, treatment can be surgical or nonsurgical. Nonsurgical treatment is typically only successful if the patient is willing to significantly modify the offending activity. Most patients do not wish to give up or modify their activities; therefore surgical treatment of chronic exertional compartment syndrome is the primary treatment. Surgical treatment is the same as an acute compartment syndrome.

However, there is debate whether fasciotomy or fasciectomy should be employed for the surgical treatment of chronic compartment syndrome. Fasciotomy, as described above, is a release or opening of the fascia allowing the compartments to be decompressed. A fasciectomy not only removes the decompressed compartment but also removes a portion of the fascia to prevent the possibility of the fascia healing back, causing recurrence of the compartment syndrome. Additionally, fasciectomy is used to treat recurrence of compartment syndrome if fasciotomy fails.

Furthermore, there is also debate on which compartments should be released. Some surgeons release only the compartment with increased pressure, whereas others release all compartments in the calf. As stated previously, the objective measures for compartment syndrome are not definitive in isolation and must be combined with the physical examination for diagnosis. With this in mind, many surgeons release all compartments due to suspicion of compartment syndrome in other compartments. This controversy is ongoing and beyond the confines of this chapter. A general guideline to follow is to release all compartments that have clinical findings consistent with compartment syndrome. The decision of which compartments to be released should also be discussed with the patient as the more compartments released increases the morbidity of the surgery and may also slow the rehabilitation.

Post-injury Equinus Contractures

Post-injury equinus contractures result from scarring of musculature in the posterior compartment of the leg. This is often the result of complications from an overlooked or unsuccessfully treated compartment syndrome. The residual scarring and contracture of the gastrocnemius and soleus from the injury lead to equinus deformity through the ankle. An equinus deformity is a plantarflexion deformity at the ankle that prevents the foot from getting to a plantigrade position when standing. This alters gate and inhibits the normal heel-to-toe motion when walking.

In addition to equinus contractures through the ankle, scarring of the deep compartment musculature can also cause clawing deformities of the toes. The deep posterior compartment of the leg is continuous with the deep calcaneal compartment in the foot. Therefore, compartment syndromes of the foot (e.g., from calcaneal fractures) can lead to a concomitant compartment syndrome of the deep posterior compartment of the leg and vice versa [8]. When an equinus contracture is noted on exam, the physician must take a detailed history to discover any previous trauma that could have caused the deformity. A thorough physical examination can identify the compartments and specific muscles involved. The Silfverskiold test should be done to determine if the equinus contracture is due to the gastrocnemius or the Achilles tendon (Fig. 10.3). This test is done with the hindfoot held in neutral and ankle dorsiflexion tested with the knee straight and also bent. Additional dorsiflexion will be noted with the knee bent if the contracture involves the gastrocnemius as it originates on the posterior femur. If operative treatment is planned to correct the deformity, an MRI can give further anatomical information as to the involved muscles and compartments.

Surgical treatment of a chronic post-injury equinus contracture will require a gastrocnemius lengthening and possibly additional tendo-Achilles lengthening. A gastrocnemius release can be done through a small incision on the posterior medial aspect of the calf centered approximately 15 cm proximal to the medial malleolus. The superficial crural fascia is split longitudinally exposing the musculotendinous junction of the gastrocnemius. After identifying and protecting the sural nerve, the gastrocnemius is released from medial to lateral just proximal to its insertion with the soleus fascia. If any residual equinus is present, the soleus fascial may be pie-crusted at this time to gain additional dorsiflexion. Pie-crusting is a technique where many small incisions in the fascia are made close to each other to allow a gradual lengthening while still maintaining the continuity of the fascia. At this point, if further release is needed, percutaneous triple hemisectioning of the Achilles tendon may be done distally to give additional lengthening. This is performed by making three small stab incisions (two medial and one lateral) with a Beaver blade centered on the Achilles tendon just proximal to its insertion. If any equinus or clawing deformities remain, the deep posterior compartment must be evaluated. This can be done by splitting the fascia longitudinally and then performing tenotomies of the involved tendons as warranted. Additionally, any scarred or nonviable tissue must be removed to establish a plantigrade foot position [3, 8]. Once surgical correction of the deformity has been completed, copious irrigation should be done and the fasciotomies left open. Skin closure can again be done with staples or nylon suture. Postoperative splinting should be used to keep the ankle in the neutral position.

Muscle Herniation (Fascial Defects)

Fascial defects can cause pain due to muscle herniation and nerve entrapment through the fascial defect. Muscle herniation can occur in any region of the lower extremity, but most often occurs

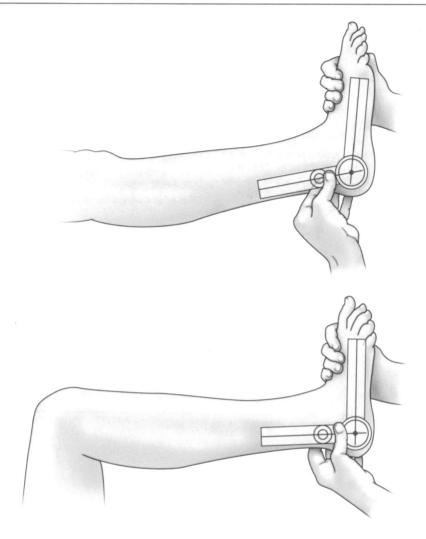

Fig. 10.3 Silfverskiold test. The ankle will have increased dorsiflexion with the knee in flexion if a gastrocnemius contracture is present

through the superficial fascia. Likewise, the most common area for nerve entrapment in the lower extremity is the superficial peroneal nerve is through the lateral compartment fascia. Undue pressure on the nerve and/or muscle causes pain. Physical exam can localize symptoms and nerve entrapment can often be detected with a positive Tinel's sign. MRI can be useful if considering surgical intervention. When identified, compartment release is indicated. Compartment release should be done in similar fashion as described above. The only alteration is that the compartment release should include the region of the fascial defect.

Summary

Most muscular injuries to the posterior lower leg can be treated nonoperatively. However, in the acute setting when function is significantly compromised or compartment syndrome occurs, surgical intervention is warranted to prevent long-term deficits. Likewise, in the chronic setting when deformities are present and function is altered, surgical intervention can restore function and rebalance the muscular forces to gain a plantigrade extremity. History and physical exam is paramount to proper diagnosis and treatment. The physician should keep a high index of suspicion for these injuries and their sequela in the lower extremity.

References

1. Perry MD, Manoli A. Foot compartment syndrome. Orthop Clin N Am. 2001;32(1):103–11.
2. Pell R, Khanuja H, Cooley R. Leg pain in the running athlete. J Am Acad Ortho Surg. 2004;12(6):396–404.
3. Manoli A, Smith DG, Hansen ST. Scarred muscle excision for the treatment of established ischemic contracture of the lower extremity. Clin Orthop. 1993;292:309–14.
4. Kirk K, Hayda R. Compartment syndrome and limb fasciotomies in the combat environment. Foot Ankle Clin N Am. 2010;15:41–61.
5. Maheshwari R, Taitsman L, Barei D. Single incision fasciotomy for compartmental syndrome of the leg in patients with diaphyseal tibia fractures. J Orthop Trauma. 2008;22(10):723–30.
6. Fraipont M, Adamson G. Chronic exertional compartment syndrome. J Am Acad Ortho Surg. 2003;11:268–76.
7. Turnipseed W, Detmer D, Girdley F. Chronic compartment syndrome. Ann Surg. 1989;210(4):557–52.
8. Perry MD, Manoli A. Reconstruction of the foot after leg or foot compartment syndrome. Foot Ankle Clin. 2006;11(1):191–201.

Rehabilitation of Injuries in the Posterior Leg

11

John Baldea, Manoj K. Dhariwal, Brock McMillen,
Casey Chrzastowski, Stacey M. Hall, Jordana Weber,
Conan Von Chittick, Premod John and Morhaf Al Achkar

Introduction

Rehabilitation of muscular injuries to the posterior lower leg encompasses a multitude of therapies, ranging from conservative cryotherapy to more invasive ultrasound-guided injection and aspiration. The treatment of these injuries often requires a team-based approach to therapy, with office-based, gym-based, and home-based rehabilitation plans. Close and frequent communication should occur between the physician, therapist, and patient. We will discuss not only muscular injuries of the posterior lower leg but also non-muscular injuries that can masquerade as a muscular injury, or otherwise complicate the clinical picture. We are presenting the most common injuries of the posterior lower leg and their corresponding rehabilitation strategies, starting with proximal anatomy and working distally. We have included a section on distal hamstring tendon injury to provide a more comprehensive regional review of the rehabilitation of injuries in the posterior leg.

Distal Hamstring Tendon Injury

While proximal and midsubstance injuries to the hamstrings are well researched and reported, little evidence exists for the management of distal hamstring tendinopathy [1–4]. Rehabilitation of

J. Baldea (✉)
Clinical Family Medicine, Indiana University School of Medicine, Family Medicine IU Health, Indianapolis, IN, USA
e-mail: jbaldea1@iuhealth.org

M. K. Dhariwal
Millennium Physician Group, Port Charlotte, FL, USA
e-mail: dhariwalmanoj@aol.com

B. McMillen
Clinical Medicine, Family Medicine, Indiana University School of Medicine—IU Methodist Hospital, Indianapolis, IN, USA
e-mail: bcmcmille@iuhealth.org

C. Chrzastowski
Outpatient Orthopedics, Rehabilitation Services, IU Health West, Avon, IN, USA
e-mail: cchrzastowsk@iuhealth.org

S. M. Hall
Physical Therapy, Indiana University Health, Indianapolis, IN, USA
e-mail: shall4@iuhealth.org

J. Weber
Family Medicine, Methodist Hospital, Indianapolis, IN, USA
e-mail: jsalamwe@iu.edu

C. Von Chittick
Family Medicine/Sports Medicine, IU Health Methodist Hospital, Indianapolis, IN, USA
e-mail: covchitt@iupui.edu

P. John
Department of Family Medicine, IU Methodist Hospital, Indianapolis, IN, USA
e-mail: pjjohn@iupui.edu

M. A. Achkar
Clinical Family Medicine, Indiana University—Methodist Hospital, Indianapolis, IN, USA
e-mail: alachkar@iupui.edu

the injured hamstring and prevention of recurrent injury should address related dysfunction in the core, pelvis, and knee as well as faulty movement patterns or athletic technique.

A phased approach to conservative outpatient rehabilitation is recommended, based on the body's healing time frame and patient-centered factors (acuity and extent of injury, mechanism of injury, level of function and type of activity, health status, and concomitant injury) [5, 6]. It is important to note that load to the tendon is the most consistent risk factor for tendinopathy identified by research and must be well managed for effective rehabilitation [6]. Factors to guide rehabilitative strategies may be inferred from the literature on hamstring injury prevention as the recurrence rate of these injuries is known to be very high.

Acuity of injury, symptoms, and functional testing should guide the patient's progression through all rehabilitative phases. It should be noted that injuries to the intramuscular portion of tendons typically result in a shorter rehabilitative period when compared to injuries that occur at the location of the muscle-free portion of the tendon [5]. The acute-phase, mid-phase, and return-to-phase rehabilitation strategies are discussed in the following sections.

If there is a true tendinitis or acute hamstring tendon tear (acute or acute-on-chronic injury), acute-phase rehabilitation begins with controlling the inflammatory process. The acronym PRICE (protect, rest, ice, compress, elevate) can be used to guide initial management. Evidence is mixed or lacking to support massage or anti-fibrotic manual therapy; electrophysical agents such as ultrasound, phonophoresis, iontophoresis, and electrical stimulation; or laser therapy in the treatment of hamstring injury [5, 7, 8]. Despite the lack of strong evidentiary support, the application of these modalities are routinely employed in the rehabilitation of soft tissue injuries (often in combination) and individualized to patient response. Future research efforts reflecting actual rehabilitation practice patterns would help inform evidence-based use of modalities.

Early mobilization within the pain-free range of motion should be initiated 2–6 days post-injury [5, 7, 9]. Therapeutic exercise with relative unloading of tendon may begin with low-intensity conditioning on a stationary bike. Lower kinetic chain and core exercises are recommended to build abdominal and gluteal strength, and may include bridges, single limb balance, and stepping agilities performed in place or in a lateral direction [5, 9, 10]. Contralateral limb exercises are suggested as there is a potential for a beneficial crossover effect (when the affected limb has improvement in muscle activation after the unaffected limb is exercised) [6]. The degree of stiffness in the passive contractile elements of antagonist muscles results in increased eccentric load on agonist muscles. Therefore, efforts to reduce passive stiffness in the quadriceps and hip flexor through stretching or other methods should result in reduced eccentric load on the hamstrings during running gait [7].

Mid-phase rehabilitation with therapeutic exercise is continued beyond the acute phase to initiate appropriate loading to the injured tendon. A strength progression for the hamstrings would include isometric to concentric to submaximal eccentric contractions. Exercises should begin in the midrange of hamstring motion and progress to more extended positions [5, 9]. Range of motion may still need to be protected, and running speed should be limited to less than 50% of the maximum to avoid damaging the recovering musculotendinous unit [5].

Specific strength exercises may be designed to address the individual muscle group injured. Since medial and lateral hamstring injuries can have different etiologies, and as the muscles may play different roles in gait and knee stabilization, it may be important to preferentially activate one muscle group [5, 11]. Beyond the early mobilization phase, stretching should be implemented in open and closed kinetic chain (CKC) positions to reestablish the length of the musculotendinous unit. Neurodynamic exercises, including sliders and tensioners, may be included if lumbar or sciatic involvement is suspected [10, 12].

General conditioning should continue to maintain the strength of the lower kinetic chain and core. Stationary biking can progress to moderate intensity. The addition of lunges, lateral shuffles, and frontal plane agilities will challenge the lower-extremity musculature and cardiovascular system without placing excessive demands on the recovering hamstrings. Continuation of gluteal and abdominal strengthening with a focus on pelvic position and control will remediate postural and motor control deficits, which may have contributed to injury. Cryotherapy is recommended after exercise sessions to manage potential pain and inflammation [5].

Return-to-function rehabilitation includes therapeutic exercises and should be designed to mimic or exceed the patient's functional demands [5, 10, 12]. Restoration of full flexibility and end-range lengthening of the muscle and tendon are the goals of stretching in this phase. Strength exercises progress to more dynamic and forceful motions with emphasis on eccentric activities [5, 6, 11]. Exercises should be multiplanar and mimic the speed and intensity of the patient's sport, work, or recreational activities.

Technique modifications for work or activity should aim to prevent reinjury and may include gait mechanics to stabilize the pelvis and prevent overstriding or postural control of the pelvic position in forward bending or the athletic ready position [9]. A functional progression should be implemented for graded exposure to sport- or work-specific tasks.

Tendinopathy of the distal hamstrings is initially managed conservatively; surgery should be reserved for patients who have failed conservative treatment of 3–6 months [3, 8, 13]. For partial tears of biceps femoris and semitendinosus tendons, conservative treatment may be attempted; however, the low success rate of conservative treatment in athletes and positive outcomes of surgical repair may make surgery a preferred option for the more active patient. Evidence-based recommendations for the conservative management of semimembranosus tendon tears are limited due to a lack of research addressing this topic. Operative outcomes were good to excellent for full semimembranosus tears, but the operative repair of partial tears carried the risk of denervation and muscle degeneration and were noted to have poor results [2].

Proximal Injuries of the Gastrocnemius and Soleus

The primary function of the gastrocnemius and soleus muscles is plantar flexion. The soleus muscle, specifically, plays an important role in maintaining posture while standing. The gastrocnemius is prone to injury because it spans the ankle and knee joints and is mostly comprised of fast-twitch muscle fibers [1]. Together, the medial and lateral heads of the gastrocnemius form an aponeurosis before integrating with the soleus muscle to form the Achilles tendon. Soleus injury is often underreported due to misdiagnosis as thrombophlebitis or the grouping of soleus strains with strains of the medial and lateral gastrocnemius muscles [14]. Mclure et al. indicated that soleus muscle strain was found to be an associated injury in 17 % of distal musculotendinous injuries to the gastrocnemius [15].

Diagnosis of proximal gastrocnemius and soleus muscle injury can normally be determined by physical examination alone. However, imaging modalities such as ultrasound and magnetic resonance imaging (MRI) are preferred to help confirm the diagnosis and determine the extent of injury if conservative rehabilitation is not progressing as expected [16].

Ultrasound may also be used to differentiate partial tears from complete tears of the muscle, which affects the rehabilitation protocol. An additional clinical use of ultrasound is to guide percutaneous aspiration of a hematoma, which is a conservative alternative to surgical intervention to relieve pressure and alleviate symptoms [17]. Ultrasound-guided aspiration of intramuscular hematomas may help to re-approximate muscle fibers and accelerate healing of an injury [17]. Ultrasound can also be used to rule out the presence of a deep-vein thrombosis, clarifying a potentially confusing clinical picture [1, 18].

Shields et al. described 25 patients who sustained an acute tear of the medial head of the gastrocnemius and were followed clinically for 1–3 years. These patients were treated without surgery, with treatment methods including a compression calf sleeve, heel lifts, and conservative outpatient rehabilitation. Eventually, these patients were advanced to calf stretches, isometric and resistance strengthening, and toe-raising exercises. The group had an average recovery time of 4.5 weeks and returned to sporting activity after an average of 6.7 weeks. After 27 months post-injury, the same group of patients underwent Cybex strength testing, which is used to evaluate extremity strength with multiple joint patterns. This testing indicated no significant differences between the injured and the non-injured limbs [18]. Kwak et al. also found that early compressive treatment in patients with injury of the medial head of the gastrocnemius decreases pain and can possibly lead to early ambulation [19].

When considering injury to the proximal gastrocnemius heads and the proximal soleus muscle, one must consider vascular structures in close proximity to these muscles, especially if conservative physical therapy or other rehabilitative treatment is not successful. The medial and lateral heads of gastrocnemius are supplied by the sural artery, which is a branch of the popliteal artery. The popliteal artery normally courses between the medial and lateral heads of the gastrocnemius muscle but may be entrapped by neighboring muscles and tendons due to variations occurring during embryonic development of the muscles and arteries [20]. Popliteal artery entrapment syndrome (PAES) is frequently seen in young males and usually presents with a complaint of intermittent calf claudication [21]. The main reason for any delay in the diagnosis of PAES is a lack of consideration for vascular pathology in patients without cardiovascular risk factors [21]. PAES will be discussed in much greater detail later in this chapter.

Kinesio Taping (KT) has become a popular treatment for rehabilitation of sports injuries and is theorized to increase circulation and subsequently improve muscle function of both the proximal gastrocnemius and soleus muscles. However, little research has been conducted to determine how KT affects athletic performance or the rehabilitation of injuries to the gastrocnemius or soleus [22, 23].

Musculotendinous Junction Injuries of the Gastrocnemius and Soleus

A partial tear of the musculotendinous junction of the medial belly of the gastrocnemius muscle is commonly referred to as tennis leg [24]. This injury usually occurs when the ankle is actively plantar flexing and the knee is extending, causing the gastrocnemius to actively contract while being passively stretched. The classic clinical picture is a middle-aged person with the complaint of an acute sports-related pain in the middle portion of the calf, generally associated with a snapping sensation [19]. A palpable gap in the muscle with calf tenderness and painful, restricted dorsiflexion may be appreciated on initial physical examination, with resolution (decrease) of the gap in time, secondary to increased calf swelling [24]. Additionally, the clinician should be aware deep venous thromboses (DVTs) often mimic muscle strains and may be associated with a muscle strain [1].

Immediate treatment for partial tears at the musculotendinous junction of the medial belly of the gastrocnemius muscle is conservative, with attention to alleviating the amount of swelling [24]. Weight bearing should be slowly increased as tolerated, and the use of crutches as well as heel lifts placed in patient's shoes may help in relieving pain [16, 24, 25]. As pain and swelling resolve, physical therapy has an important role in facilitating recovery, with early interventions including gentle calf stretching, massage, and cryotherapy [25, 26]. As the acute symptoms resolve, strength training, proprioception training, heel raises, and closed-chain exercises are then added along with core strengthening and general conditioning [26]. According to Toulipolous et al., most patients who receive conservative treatment fully recover and have a low rate of recurrence. Even in cases of large tears, conservative treatment is recommended, given that repair of the musculotendinous junction is not shown to produce superior results to nonoperative care [25]. With regard to a time frame for return to pre-injury-activity levels, Perkins et al. note that ambulation without pain may take 2–12 weeks post-injury [24]; furthermore, Kwak et al. note that healing of a muscle rupture occurs slowly and may take upwards of 3–16 weeks [27].

Therapies already referenced in this section for the rehabilitation of proximal gastrocnemius injuries can also be applied to more distal musculotendinous injuries. Kwak et al. concluded that early compression therapy may lead to earlier ambulation as well as decreasing the amount of fluid collection after rupture of the medial head of the gastrocnemius. This study suggests that patients with muscle rupture during exercise or training should be treated with early compression, ice, and immobilization to limit acute hemorrhage [27].

Injury to the soleus is uncommon and rarely reported [1]. According to Campbell, when looking at the statistics from 141 patients who were referred for ultrasound examination following a calf strain, 67% had tears to the gastrocnemius, 21% had hematoma and fluid accumulation but no definitive muscle tear, 9% had deep vein thrombosis, 1.4% had a plantaris rupture, and 0.7% had an isolated soleus tear [26]. Injury to this muscle may be underrepresented due to misdiagnosis as a tear or strain of the gastrocnemius or as thrombophlebitis [1, 16]. Soleus muscle strain was found to be associated with upwards of 17% of distal musculotendinous injuries to the gastrocnemius [1, 16].

The soleus is considered at low risk for injury as compared to the gastrocnemius; furthermore, the clinical presentation of soleus strains is generally less dramatic and more sub-acute in comparison to gastrocnemius injuries [16]. Soleus injury may present as calf tightness, stiffness, and pain, which is exacerbated by walking or jogging and worsens over days to weeks [16].

As the prevalence of soleus injuries are minimal when compared to other posterior leg injuries, and at times are found in conjunction with gastrocnemius injuries, their treatment is much like the aforementioned rehabilitation of medial gastrocnemius injuries. In general, when taking into account any calf strain, an accurate diagnosis as well as early appropriate treatment can significantly affect duration and amount of disability [16]. Similar to the goals of treatment of medial gastrocnemius rupture/strain, acute treatment of soleus injury should be aimed at limiting hemorrhage and pain as well as preventing complications [16]. According to Dixon, during the first 3–5 days, rest is achieved by limiting stretching and contraction; in addition, it is recommended to utilize cryotherapy, compressive wrap or tape, and elevation of the leg. While nonsteroidal anti-inflammatory drugs (NSAIDs) should be restricted for the first 24–72 h due to their antiplatelet effect (increased bleeding), Celebrex and other COX-2 inhibitors may be an option due to their lack of antiplatelet effect. Dixon advises against moist heat and massage early in the healing process because these treatments are thought to increase the risk of hemorrhage [16].

More active rehabilitation may follow successful acute treatment. Rehabilitative exercises should isolate affected muscles (gastrocnemius versus soleus) by varying the degree of knee flexion. Passive stretching should ensue during the sub-acute phase to help elongate the maturing intermuscular scar as well as prepare the muscle for strengthening. According to Dixon, once the range of motion returns, unloaded isometric contractions are recommended to begin strengthening. Therapeutic exercise selection should progress by sequentially introducing pain-free isometric, isotonic, and then dynamic training exercises, thereby controlling the variables that affect strain on the injured tissue [16].

Popliteus

As the popliteus is a smaller structure with limited function in the posterior lower leg, the incidence of injury is much lower than other larger structures. Thus, the available literature on rehabilitation of popliteus injuries is limited. The popliteus muscle's primary action is to medially rotate the tibia on the femur and prevent tibial external rotation, but it also helps to prevent forward displacement of the femur on the tibia when standing on a partially flexed knee [28–30]. The popliteus muscle is a significant component to 3D stability of the knee joint complex, including transverse-plane rotation of the long axis of the tibia and femur. Individual differences in static standing tibia and femoral rotation are components of genu varus and genu valgus postures. Therefore, it is important to consider the hip joint controlling abduction or adduction of the femur in the frontal plane and the subtalar joint controlling supination and pronation [28, 31].

The acute phase of healing in a popliteus muscle strain is essential as this is when blood is being distributed to the area to bring nutrients and stimulate new growth [31]. There is increased debate over the role of therapeutic ultrasound to encourage the healing process of an injured muscle or tendon. As a general treatment approach to musculotendinous injuries, Fu et al. found that low-intensity pulsed ultrasound, if utilized within the first 2 weeks of an injury, could help promote tendon healing [32]. Cryotherapy and compression with a knee sleeve could also help decrease pain and edema that may occur in the popliteal fossa. Prolonged immobilization should be avoided following a muscle strain, for example of the popliteus, to prevent the potential for increased stiffness [33]. It is also important to maintain range of motion (ROM) and strength of adjacent joints, with the greatest focus being on restoring and maintaining anatomical alignment [31].

When pain and swelling have been controlled, the body has begun the repair–regeneration stage of healing, where new collagen is being distributed to rebuild the damaged tissue [31]. It is during this phase that it is important to avoid overloading the tissue. Any increased signs in warmth, edema, and pain are signs the load is too great [31]. Isometric exercises are described as a proprioceptive neuromuscular technique to increase strength and stability at particular portions through the range of motion. This technique is most effective for the popliteus at varying degrees of tibial internal rotation within a 0–30° knee flexion range [31].

During the return to sport phase of healing, CKC exercises can be utilized to stimulate co-contractions that promote dynamic stabilization, improving postural support for the joint [31]. Utilizing CKC exercises can stimulate the proprioceptive system to improve balance and stability. Nyland et al. suggest a series of dynamic stepping lunges in a cross-body pattern, incorporating various degrees of tibial rotation (Fig. 11.1) [28]. The result of this type of plyometric training is improved neuromuscular control and increased tolerance to stretch loads [31]. Pyometric

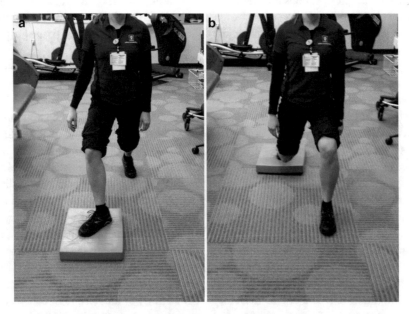

Fig. 11.1 Dynamic stepping lunges. The lunge begins with slow controlled eccentric loading (**a**), followed by explosive concentric contraction to return to the starting position (**b**)

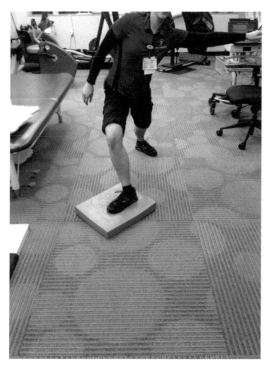

Fig. 11.2 Single-limb lunge stance with lateral reach

exercises should be initiated in a single plane (Fig. 11.2) and then progress to include the 3D stability component (Fig. 11.3) [31]. To further challenge the patient, catching and tossing weighted balls will increase the specificity of the

task. The addition of the weighted ball toss also redirects the patients' attention, allowing true assessment of their ability to maintain the 3D stance. Having the patient close their eyes or adding a compliant surface under the stance limb further challenges the proprioceptive system. When the patient is able to maintain a level pelvis and subtalar neutral position with the above lunge positions, incorporating small jumps progressing toward a bounding motion will assist in progression toward dynamic athletic activity.

Neurovascular Entrapment

Neurovascular entrapment, including diagnoses such as PAES, can occur when the popliteal artery and other neurovascular structures become compressed between muscles and tendons in the posterior lower leg due to variations in embryonic development [20]. The main reason for delay in diagnosis of neurovascular entrapment is a lack of consideration for vascular or neurological pathology in patients without cardiovascular risk factors [21].

Use of neurodynamic mobilization as a treatment for neurovascular entrapment has become increasingly popular in the rehabilitation of this disorder. Prolonged compression of a nerve can

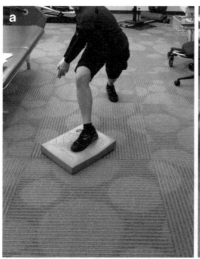
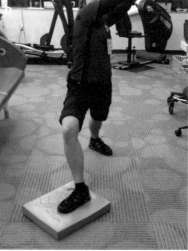

Fig. 11.3 Single-limb stance and reaching with contralateral trunk rotation

lead to edema and increased pressure, resulting in additional compression due to intraneural thickening. It has been demonstrated that neurodynamic mobilization techniques can reduce intraneural edema and decrease the effects of compression from surrounding fascial restrictions [34]. Neural mobilization techniques increase excursion by "flossing" the nerve. This technique attempts to mobilize the neural tissue both proximally and then distally [35]. Alternating between elongating and shortening the nerve creates a pumping effect to help decrease edema by dispersing the intraneural fluid [34]. It has been suggested that these mobilization techniques should be performed in a slow and rhythmic fashion to prevent excessive strain, which would in turn inhibit blood flow and further damage the nerve.

It is also important to evaluate the location of the injury and consider joint position during these mobilization techniques. Boyd et al. discuss the effects of proximal–distal sequencing versus a distal–proximal sequencing of joint movement to create neural gliding [36]. The joint closest to the injured site is more irritable due to intraneural edema and, therefore, should remain somewhat stationary, given that the greatest amount of strain occurs at the moving joint [35, 36]. Butler et al. describe varying techniques for passive and active mobilization strategies for the tibial and peroneal nerves [37]. A combination of ankle dorsiflexion and eversion with knee extension and hip flexion provides maximal elongation of the tibial nerve. For the sural nerve, maximal elongation comes from a combination of ankle dorsiflexion and inversion with knee extension and hip flexion [37].

Mobilizing the nerve through surrounding structures is a key component of the rehabilitation process, but consideration of the fascial restrictions causing the entrapment is critical. Addressing these restrictions with myofascial release techniques has been found to be beneficial as a conservative management [37]. Moreover, consideration of why these restrictions may be present through assessment of an anatomical alignment is important in rehabilitation for prevention of recurrence [37]. The final stage of rehabilitation should consist of developing a home exercise program to increase tissue extensibility of restricted muscles and to strengthen weak muscles that may contribute to any postural misalignments [37].

Tibialis Posterior

Tibialis posterior injuries are a very common problem in sports medicine. Although they are rarely reported or studied, posterior tibialis tendon issues are a common cause of acquired adult flat foot, among other problems, and the mechanism of injury has not been clearly elucidated [38].

Musculoskeletal abnormalities can usually be diagnosed by the use of the mnemonic "TART": Tenderness, Asymmetry, Restricted motion, and Tissue texture abnormality [39]. Dixon et al. described a three-grade classification of calf muscle strains based on disability, physical findings, and pathologic correlation. Although there is consensus about the use of a three-grade classification, there seems to be disagreement in the semantics of the grading system [16]. Johnson and Strom described a classification for tibialis posterior tendon insufficiency classification, later complemented by Myerson [38, 40]. Although this is a grading system for tendon insufficiency and not muscular strain, Howitt et al. considers the three-stage Johnson and Strom system useful for establishing treatment strategies as the acute tibialis posterior strain would be equivalent to a stage 1 or 2 of this classification scale [38].

There seems to be consensus regarding the initial treatment of acute muscle strain. Similar to prior sections of this chapter, most experts agree about the inclusion of the PRICE system for initial management of tibialis posterior muscle strains, as with any other muscle strains [16, 38–40]. Symptom control, avoidance of hemorrhage, and other complications should be the main goals of this phase [16, 38].

Protection from further injury must be one of the initial steps. Only severe injuries require total immobilization and avoidance of weight-bearing [39, 41]. Use of braces or other orthotic devices are particularly useful to correct biomechanical problems, which may hinder optimal healing [42]. Rest with a relative limitation of physical activity, decreased repetitive loading, and cessation of participation in sports for a short period of time as determined by the severity of the symptoms might be needed to achieve symptom control and prevent further injuries [39, 42]. A brief period of immobilization, usually limited to no more than 1 week, is recommended to allow the scar tissue to gain the necessary strength to tolerate the forces applied over the new tissue; this will have the beneficial effect of preventing acute reinjuries and retraction of the muscle stump [43]. Prolonged immobilization should be avoided if possible to prevent muscular atrophy and deconditioning [42].

Cryotherapy by applying ice to the affected area intermittently has been recommended in multiple studies. It has been effective for short-duration pain relief and swelling control. It has also been associated with smaller hematomas between the myofiber stumps [43]. Although there is agreement in the general effectiveness of cryotherapy, there is no consensus regarding the specific duration and interval of the therapy. Some authors recommend intermittent application for a 10 min duration, while others recommend periods of 15–20 min [39, 42, 43]. Recent research suggests the greatest benefit of cryotherapy occurs in the 6 h following the initial trauma [43].

Compression is a component of the PRICE treatment and has been widely recommended in several studies in combination with cryotherapy at similar intervals because it reduces blood flow to the injured fibers. However, there is no conclusive information regarding the use of compression in the acute phase of the injury, and it has not been proven to hasten healing [16, 38, 39, 43].

Elevation is also used in combination with the other components of PRICE as it decreases the hydrostatic pressure when elevating the injury above the heart, thus decreasing the potential for local edema [43].

NSAIDs have been recommended for inflammation and pain control [38, 41]. Some authors recommend that NSAID use should be restricted during the first 24–72 h due to potential worsening of hemorrhage as a result of anticoagulant effects, but Celecoxib and other COX-2 selective inhibitors might be an option as they do not affect platelets [16, 38]. Other authors recommend limiting the use of NSAIDs to a short-term period during the early stages of healing as they decrease the inflammatory reaction without affecting the healing process or myofiber regeneration [43]. The same study recommends short-term use because long-term use might have an effect on the regeneration of skeletal muscle. Acetaminophen and narcotics may be used as well to help control pain [16, 44]. Alternatively, the use of topical NSAIDs might reduce pain with less risk of gastrointestinal complications.

The use of corticosteroids has been controversial in musculotendinous lesions. Glucocorticoids have led to retardation of tissue regeneration as well as delayed elimination of hematomas and necrotic tissue [43, 45]. Based on the literature, use of glucocorticoids appears to lead to an increase in the strength of affected and non-affected muscles during the initial 2 days of healing versus control groups. However, after 1 week of treatment, injured and non-injured muscles showed weakness when compared to control groups. Alternately, muscular injuries treated with anabolic steroids showed no differences during the first 2 days when compared to controls, but the group treated with anabolic steroids showed an increase in the strength of the injured muscle after 1 week of treatment when compared with the contralateral muscle and with the control group [45].

Therapeutic ultrasound has been widely recommended for the acute treatment of muscular injuries. Typical parameters in application of therapeutic ultrasound for this indication would be a 50% duty cycle with 1 MHz frequency and 0.7 W intensity, with a duration of between 5 and 15 min. It has been proposed that therapeutic ultrasound, performed within the parameters listed above, could enhance the initial stage of muscular regeneration [43]. However, several studies have found that there is no improvement in healing time when compared with non-treated muscle injuries. Aside from the analgesic effect of the high-frequency ultrasound waves, there is no other additional benefit of ultrasound therapy [43, 46].

Manual therapy techniques are often employed in the rehabilitation of soft tissue injuries. Although many approaches to manual therapy exist, Active Release Techniques® (ART®), Graston Technique®, and Astym® are some of the most popular applications of manual therapy in rehabilitation settings. In ART®, deep digital tension is applied at the affected area, and the patient moves actively through identified sites of soft tissues adhesions from a shortened to a lengthened position. This modality of therapy requires knowledge of the anatomy of the limbs and comprehension of the traversing tissues located at angles. It has been used in cases of tibialis posterior strains with adequate results [38]. Graston Technique®, a form of instrument-assisted tissue mobilization, uses patented stainless steel instruments with beveled edges that are used to manipulate and mobilize the tissue with the goal of decreasing fascia irregularities. The Graston Technique® is based on the belief that treatment in this way will enhance proliferation of extracellular matrix fibroblasts, improve ion transport, and decrease cell matrix adhesions. Astym® also uses a specialized instrument set to mobilize soft tissue by transferring pressure and sheer force to the underlying dysfunctional soft tissue with the goal of increasing fibroblast recruitment and tissue quality.

Experimental studies initially showed that hyperbaric oxygen, or HBO, accelerated the recovery of injured skeletal muscle in animals. However, more recent meta-analysis has shown that HBO might actually increase the sensation of pain in milder degrees of muscular injury [43]. The use of HBO for skeletal muscle injuries is rare and remains experimental.

Although there is plenty of literature indicating the destruction of sarcomeres and muscular damage secondary to eccentric exercises, it has been proposed that a mild eccentric exercise program might protect the muscle from further damage due to adaptation of the sarcomeres, therefore leading to fewer areas of potential instability [47]. The role of eccentric exercise in acute soft tissue injury rehabilitation remains antithetical, and additional investigation would be needed prior to application in the initial phase of a rehabilitation program.

The goal of the sub-acute and chronic phases of tibialis posterior injuries should be directed toward the modification of training regimens and correcting the mechanics of the lower leg as well as training errors [39]. As the muscle fails progressively, the calcaneus rotates into a valgus angle, the arch collapses, and the forefoot gradually abducts, likely producing an acquired flat foot [40]. A key part of the treatment is assessing the need for adequate footwear with shock-absorbing soles and insoles that might fix easily correctable problems. It is also recommended to change shoes every 250–500 miles [39–41]. The use of lace-up shoes is generally recommended to improve foot stabilization. Some patients might be able to correct issues with off-the-shelf orthotics [38–40].

After the acute phase of rehabilitation, the athlete may begin gradually exercising as tolerated. Runners or triathletes may start swimming and cycling, and tibialis posterior strengthening exercises such as heel-ups with a tennis ball held between the medial malleoli can be initiated (Fig. 11.4) [38]. To avoid complete cessation of activities, a 50% decrease in the weekly running distance, frequency, and intensity may also be recommended to runners for a period of 2–6 weeks. Running on uneven surfaces should initially be avoided, and a synthetic track or other uniform surface of moderate firmness may provide more shock absorption [39]. Running on un-

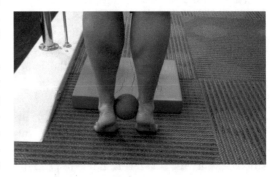

Fig. 11.4 Heel-ups with a tennis ball

even surfaces may then be gradually introduced and progressed as tolerated [44].

The decision to start return to sport-specific practices can be made after two conditions have been met: First, the athlete must be able to stretch the injured muscle as much as the contralateral side; additionally, the athlete must be able to perform pain-free basic movements with the injured muscle. If both conditions have been met, the athlete may start training gradually, preferably under the supervision of an athletic trainer [43].

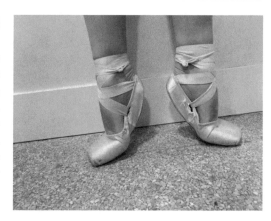

Fig. 11.5 Ballet position—demi-pointe

Flexor Hallucis Longus

Flexor hallucis longus (FHL) injury is the most common lower extremity tendinitis in classical ballet dancers and is sometimes referred to as "dancer's tendonitis." This injury is also seen in persons who participate in activities requiring frequent push-off maneuvers and extreme plantar flexion, such as swimmers, ice skaters, long-distance runners, and gymnasts [48, 49]. As flexor hallicus longus injuries are most common in dancers, the rehabilitation techniques in this section are geared primarily toward helping dancers but can be adapted for other individuals.

In dancers, the FHL tendon is generally stressed in the direction of overlengthening as it functions as a medial stabilizer of the ankle in the externally rotated position of the lower limb known as the dancer's "turnout." Prevention can be the best form of treatment. FHL injuries can be prevented by reducing turnout of the hip, so the dancer is working directly over the foot. Additional training techniques to help prevent FHL injuries include: avoiding en pointe exercises and hard floors whenever possible, gripping of the floor with the toes when jumping, strengthening the body's core, and wearing firm, well-fitted shoes. Prehabilitation exercises to improve ankle stability, such as proprioception exercises (wobble board, TheraBand) should be encouraged [49–51].

For post-injury rehabilitation, the focus should be on correction of muscle imbalances, weakness, and faulty technique as mainstays of treatment. For dancers, correction of "over-turning out" should be the first-line treatment, as well as strengthening the anti-pronation muscles of the ankle and the intrinsic muscles of the foot to support the medial longitudinal arch. A careful examination will establish whether there are faults in technique. In conjunction with technique correction, strengthening of the hip and core musculature to support the correct turnout technique is important.

Dancers can relatively unload the flexor hallucis longus tendon during healing by avoiding work on demi-pointe (end-range weight-bearing plantar flexion; Fig. 11.5) and full pointe (Fig. 11.6), and by minimizing jumping due to push-off demands. Optimal floor cushioning would theoretically help to reduce tendon overload, but hard floors in the studio are unfortunately impossible to avoid. In addition, injuries can arise from floors that are too soft or from any rapid change in training surface, so caution should be advised in modifying the training surface. Moreover, dancers are required to wear minimal footwear in the studio (ballet slippers, pointe shoes, etc.), and changing their footwear to rest an injury is next to impossible during participation. However, use of supportive shoes outside of class is a reasonable expectation [52].

Most authors recommend 6 months of nonsurgical treatment prior to consideration of surgical intervention for flexor hallucis longus injuries. Unfortunately, reported failure rates for nonoperative management range from 40 to 100%. Common treatment approaches include rest, administration

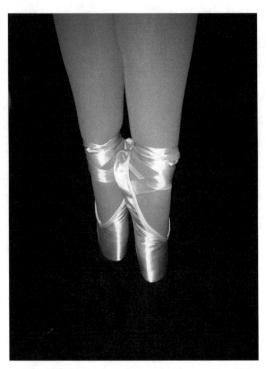

Fig. 11.6 Ballet position—full pointe

of NSAID medications, ice or contrast baths, gentle stretching, massage, water therapy, and ultrasound [51].

One of the more successful nonoperative treatments is the FHL stretch exercise. To perform this exercise, the patient stands facing the wall with a book placed under the hallux. While keeping the heel on the ground, the ankle is maximally dorsiflexed by flexing the knee. Typically, the stretching is performed for 30 s, repeated three to five times. A more limited protocol of stretching 10 s for ten repetitions with each set of stretches being repeated three to four times daily may be helpful as a general gliding mobilization of the tendon [53].

Stretching, however, is not always an effective treatment because the tissue is often overlengthened and too painful. If stretching aggravates or fails to improve symptoms, immobilization in a walking boot is often necessary. Initially, the walking boot can be used at night for 6 weeks. If symptoms fail to diminish, use of a walking boot (or application of a short leg walking cast

extending past the toes) should be applied full time for 6 weeks. If a walking boot is used for immobilization, it can be combined with intermittent use of the FHL stretching exercise as tolerated. After 6 weeks of walking boot use, the patient should progress to a full program of FHL stretching and a formal rehabilitation program as outlined above [49–51].

Intra-tendinous injections of steroids in the FHL, as in all forms of tendinitis, should be avoided because of the risk of weakening or rupturing of the tendon. Ultrasound-guided injection of corticosteroids into the flexor hallucis longus tendon sheath vastly decreases the risk of tendon rupture and has led to clinical success in the experience of the senior author of this chapter. If triggering of the tendon is present, or symptoms are unresponsive to 6 months of conservative treatment, surgical decompression and repair of the tendon may be necessary [51, 53].

Chronic Exertional Compartment Syndrome

Chronic exertional compartment syndrome , or CECS, can occur in any compartment of the extremities, although the leg is the most common location [54].

Conservative treatment is frequently attempted for CECS; however, typically, it has been thought to be generally unsuccessful for athletes who wish to train or compete at a high level. Conservative management generally involves a decrease in activity or load to the affected compartment. This effectively results in detraining of the muscles within the effected compartment and can reduce compartment pressures. After detraining, activity level is gradually increased and titrated based on the patient's symptoms. During detraining, cross-training exercises like swimming, bicycling, and other low-impact activities are prescribed. Aquatic exercises, such as running in water, are often employed to maintain fitness while improving mobility and strength without unnecessarily loading the affected compartment. Massaging and stretching exercises have also been shown to be occasionally effective in CECS.

In addition to activity modification, biomechanical correction with orthotics and the use of NSAID medications are often prescribed. Pain control with analgesics may be warranted in patients with CECS for acute symptom management, but they play a minimal role in the treatment of this condition. It is generally recommended to avoid compression of the affected limb as this may result in increased compartment pressures. Some athletes have symptoms that are worse on certain surfaces (concrete versus running track or artificial turf versus grass) and symptoms may be relieved by switching surfaces [55].

It should be noted that the presence of muscle weakness in CECS does not necessarily indicate the need for a muscle strengthening program. Exercise brings on the symptoms of CECS and leads to hypertrophy of the muscles within the compartment; therefore, muscle strengthening is problematic for these patients. Only patients with very mild CECS may be able to build strength without precipitating abnormal compartment pressures [56].

Research has suggested that treatment with anti-inflammatory medications, stretching, prolonged rest, ultrasound, electrical stimulation, orthotics, and massage have resulted in limited success, but assessing and correcting biomechanical faults is a core component of rehabilitation for CECS. For example, a hindfoot strike gait pattern leads to increase ground-reaction forces, stride length, and ground-contact time. Thus, it is possible that training and adopting a forefoot running technique may be effective in reducing the symptoms of athletes with CECS who hindfoot strike by adopting a forefoot running technique [57].

Despite the limitations described above, a trial of conservative treatment should be undertaken for most patients with CECS. Along with activity modification, this should include gait analysis, biomechanical correction, and a trial of gait retraining. If conservative therapy is unsuccessful, the patient should be referred for compartment pressure testing and surgical consultation for consideration of release of the effected compartments [55].

Achilles Tendon

Achilles tendon, the largest and strongest tendon in the body, connects the calcaneus to the gastrocnemius and soleus muscles. Due to its function and limited blood supply, the tendon is vulnerable to injury that is difficult to heal. Common pathologies of the Achilles tendon include tendinitis, peritendonitis, tendinosis, and rupture. These conditions are generally caused by overuse and can occur in adolescents and adults.

Cryotherapy is regarded as the single most effective modality for tendon inflammation, with sufficient evidence throughout the literature. An Achilles tendon injury, like any other injury to the body, initiates a cascade of normal inflammatory physiology. During an injury, vasodilatation leads to capillary permeability with fluid extravasation and swelling, metabolic changes, and increased pro-inflammatory cytokines. Cryotherapy combined with compression therapy has been shown to decrease microcirculation at the mid-portion of the Achilles tendon space, promoting preservation of deep tendon oxygen saturation and facilitated venous capillary outflow [58].

Another therapeutic modality, phonophoresis, harnesses the acoustic effects of ultrasound to assist in driving medications into tissue. Acoustic stimuli produce four distinct effects on tissue: thermal, non-thermal, neural, and connected effects. Thermal effects coincide with the absorption of sound energy, and the corresponding heat can be augmented by the increase in frequency; 90 kHz of ultrasound can penetrate tissue to a depth of 10 cm. Non-thermal effects are due to acoustic pressure changes within the tissue, which can be used to help propel medications into soft tissue. Ultrasound also stimulates increased fibroblast activity and increases dispensability of tissues [59].

Iontophoresis is another therapeutic modality for the treatment of Achilles tendinopathy. This modality uses electric stimulation to produce an electric field between two electrodes and uses ions from medication to diffuse through tissue. Iontophoresis is contraindicated for individuals who have a pacemaker, are pregnant, are diabetic, have electrical hypersensitivity, or have skin allergies. Although the patient population was small, a double-blind study reported positive results when iontophoresis was used with dexamethasone as compared to iontophoresis with saline solution. Following treatment with iontophoresis, both groups participated in a rehabilitation program in which 10 participants were followed up at 3, 6, and 12 months. Although both groups noted improvement of Achilles pain during the length of the study, the group with iontophoresis and dexamethasone reported less pain while walking at 3, 6, and 12 months [60].

Since the mid-1980s, eccentric loading exercises have been a mainstay in the treatment of Achilles tendinopathy. Curwin and Standish demonstrated successful resolution of symptoms with a simple 6-week program of progressive eccentric tendon load [61]. In 1998, Alfredson et al. developed a model for eccentric calf muscle training to the point of provoked pain at the Achilles tendon. The muscles are loaded with the knee straight and, to maximize the activation of the soleus muscle, also with the knee bent. The patient stands with their forefoot on the edge of a step or curb with the ankle joint in full plantar flexion (Fig. 11.7a). The patient slowly lowers himself or herself into full dorsiflexion using the affected limb only (Fig. 11.7b). At this point, the uninjured leg should be used to reposition the patient back to the starting point.

The patient should be able to perform the eccentric loading to the point of provoking pain. Treatment should be stopped if the patient begins to have disabling pain. If performing the loading technique with body weight alone does not provoke pain, a weighted backpack should be used [62, 64]. Eccentric training should be performed twice daily, 7 days a week, for 12 weeks. Follow-up studies have shown a decrease in thickness and volume as well as a change in the neovascularization of the Achilles tendon after eccentric loading [63–66].

After a tendon injury, a histopathological response takes place within the damaged tendon. Chronic tendinopathy can lead to degradation and synthesis of the cell matrix in response to different stressors [67]. This process stimulates connective tissue remodeling through resorption and synthesis of collagen secondary to fibroblast recruitment [68]. Assisted manual therapy techniques are often employed in the rehabilitation of chronic tendinopathy to attempt to address these changes. Although many approaches to instrument-assisted manual therapy exist, Graston Technique® and Astym® are currently two of the most popular applications. The Graston

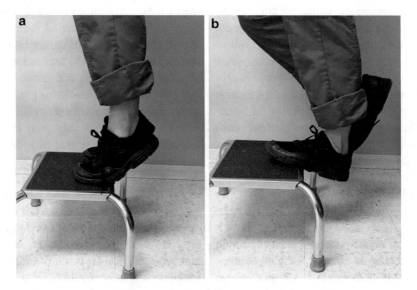

Fig. 11.7 Alfredson model for eccentric calf muscle training to the point of provoked pain at the Achilles tendon. **a** Full plantar flexion. **b** Full dorsiflexion

Technique® employs patented stainless steel instruments with beveled edges that are used to manipulate and mobilize the tissue with the goal of decreasing fascia irregularities, enhancing proliferation of extracellular matrix fibroblasts, improve ion transport, and decrease cell matrix adhesions. Astym® also uses a specialized instrument set to mobilize soft tissue by transferring pressure and sheer force to the underlying dysfunctional soft tissue. Astym® moves along the direction of the underlying tissue, in contrast to cross-frictional techniques, which apply transverse pressure to the underlying tissue. Specially designed instruments are used in a stroking motion along the skin while using a lubricant, such as cocoa butter, to reduce the coefficient of friction. This stroking motion along the underlying tissue increases fibroblast recruitment and activation in animal studies but has not been thoroughly studied in humans [69].

Retrocalcaneal Bursitis

Retrocalcaneal bursitis is inflammation of the bursa in the recess between the anterior inferior side of the Achilles tendon and the posterior superior aspect of the calcaneus [70]. Acute rehabilitation for retrocalcaneal bursitis should have a methodical approach, including the previously mentioned PRICE therapy, anti-inflammatory medications, ultrasound, and electrical stimulation [71]. Initial treatment should focus on reduction of pressure to the area with open-back shoes, using heel lifts, orthotic devices, or rocker sole shoes to reduce pressure on the Achilles tendon and bursa [71, 72]. The use of orthotics and specialized shoes focuses on reduction of direct pressure on the retrocalcaneal space. It is recommended that, after the resolution of symptoms, patients carefully select their shoe type based on the amount of pressure exerted on the retrocalcaneal area. Caution is also advised at the selection of orthotics for the correction of foot plane deformities so that they are not overcorrected, particularly in runners [73]. It should be noted that some data suggest that orthotic insoles do not decrease the rate of lower limb overuse injuries such as retrocalcaneal bursitis [74].

In general, the use of injectable steroids in this area is contraindicated as it may lead to tendon rupture; however, in refractory cases of retrocalcaneal bursitis, a one-time steroid injection directly into the retrocalcaneal bursa is sometimes helpful [75].

Posterior Impingement Syndrome

Posterior impingement syndrome occurs during full weight bearing in full plantar flexion and can be caused by a variety of problems including an os trigonum (Fig. 11.8), Steida process, arthritis, or FHL tendinitis/tenosynovitis [76, 77]. It has been reported that conservative care is successful in 60% of patients with posterior impingement syndrome [78, 79]. In cases where conservative care fails to resolve pain and function, arthroscopic surgery is recommended to remove the excessive bony prominences, release and/or debride tendons, or repair torn tendons [77, 79]. Rehabilitation is key for both conservative and postoperative recovery from posterior impingement syndrome.

Acute rehabilitation of posterior impingement syndrome should include restriction or modification of activity, especially activities that cause or increase pain. Use of NSAIDs, steroid injections, ice, elevation, compression, and possibly immobilization in a short leg boot for those with severe symptoms has also been reported by several authors [79, 80]. Physical therapy recommendations include initiating gentle stretching of the gastrocnemius, soleus and FHL; joint mobilizations; and gentle strengthening of the lower leg muscles, including the deep foot muscles involved in plantar flexion and ankle isometrics [78, 81]. Pain-free cross-training activities such as stationary bicycling or aquatic therapy are also initiated [82].

Mid-phase rehabilitation focuses on joint mobility throughout the foot and ankle, and flexibility in the entire lower-extremity functional chain. Strengthening should focus on medial and

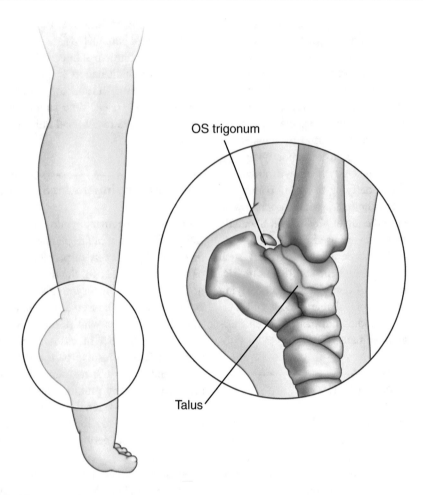

Fig. 11.8 Os trigonum syndrome

lateral control throughout the entire range of motion from dorsiflexion to full plantarflexion in both open- and closed-chain activities, as well as deceleration strength of the ankle dorsiflexors for managing dynamic stability in terminal plantarflexion. Proprioceptive exercises are initiated to improve lower-extremity biomechanics and stability [80, 83]. Ankle, foot, knee, or pelvic malalignments are also corrected in this phase to prepare for return to function [84, 85].

Return-to-function rehabilitation encompasses stretching and strengthening, which continues from the previous phases with increasing difficulty. The patient is slowly transitioned back into his or her activities through functional sports progressions.

Significant efforts are undertaken in retraining and technique modification for sport-specific activities. Many authors state that technique faults and/or compensations for poor flexibility, weakness, and poor mobility contribute to increased risk for (re)injury. Correction of these faults and compensations is vital in preventing further injury. A comprehensive lower-extremity and core strengthening program with a neuromuscular re-education program to correct any compensatory strategies is essential to return to full activity without recurrence of symptoms [83, 85].

If symptoms do not resolve with conservative care, arthroscopic surgery is recommended, followed by physical therapy focusing on ROM, progressive strengthening and stretching, and return to function as described above [86, 87].

Sever's Apophysitis

Calcaneal apophysitis is a common cause of heel pain in children, most often in those who participate in sports such as soccer, basketball, track, and other running or closed-chain impact activities. Once thought to be an overuse traction injury creating inflammation at the apophysis, due to recent imaging techniques and studies, it is now believed to be an overuse compression injury leading to microfracture of the calcaneal apophysis [81, 88–90].

In acute-phase rehabilitation, patients take a brief period of rest from the aggravating activities. Patients are rarely immobilized, except for cases of severe and extreme pain. Modified and pain-free activities are encouraged, including cross-training exercises that do not aggravate symptoms, such as swimming and stationary bicycling. Patients are also advised to use ice, NSAIDs, and elevation to alleviate pain. Heel lifts or cushions are beneficial in helping to relieve symptoms. Ice, heat, iontophoresis with dexamethasone sodium phosphate, and Ketoprofen gel has been used in the management of pain with some success [90, 91].

Mid-phase rehabilitation is recommended to provide instruction and supervised exercises and activities to restore flexibility, strength, and function. Such activities include stretching of the gastrocnemius and soleus complex, hamstrings, quadriceps, and all other muscles found to be deficient in flexibility in the lower-extremity kinetic chain. Strengthening of the ankle dorsiflexors and other foot and ankle muscles is also initiated in mid-phase rehabilitation. Full lower-extremity strengthening in both the open and CKC is initiated, as tolerated by pain, in order to maintain functional chain strength. Proprioception exercises are also initiated, if tolerated, to prepare for return to sport/function training [85, 91].

With return-to-function rehabilitation, the therapist will continue stretching the lower-extremity kinetic chain, both static and dynamic, although static stretching has been found to provide better gains in flexibility than dynamic stretching [91]. Strengthening of the kinetic chain continues with progression to impact-type closed-chain exercises and activities that address specific weaknesses in the lower extremity and core. Progressions to dynamic proprioceptive activities that are more sport-specific are introduced. Once the patient is pain-free, functional sports progressions, especially for running, are initiated. Training to correct sport-specific techniques is crucial in rehabilitation and return to sport, especially to prevent reinjury. Correction of improper running and jumping techniques is crucial to prevent recurrence of symptoms [85, 91].

Conclusion

The rehabilitation of injuries to the posterior leg is multifaceted and often aided by the clinical and basic science literature. It is imperative that close and frequent communication occurs between patient, physician, and rehabilitation professionals. This team-based approach to treatment is particularly important for posterior leg injuries as the diagnosis can be difficult, and options for treatment often include specialized services that are multidisciplinary in nature. We have presented a review of injuries to the posterior leg and a discussion of corresponding rehabilitation plans. We hope that this will be a valuable resource to support your evaluation and treatment of patients with muscular injuries to the posterior leg.

References

1. Armfield DR, Kim DH-M, et al. Sports-related muscle injury in the lower extremity. Clin Sports Med. 2006;25(4):803–42.
2. Lempainen L, Sarimo J, Mattila K, et al. Distal tears of the hamstring muscles: review of the literature and our results of surgical treatment. Br J Sports Med. 2007;41(2):80–3.
3. Bylund WE, de Weber K. Semimembranosus tendinopathy: one cause of chronic posteromedial knee pain. Sports. 2010;2(5):380–4.
4. Ropiak CR, Bosco JA. Hamstring injuries. Bull NYU Hosp Jt Dis. 2012;70(1):41–8.
5. Heiderscheidt BC, Sherry MA, Silder A, et al. Hamstring strain injuries: recommendations for diagnosis, rehabilitation and injury prevention. J Orthop Sports Phys Ther. 2010;40(2):67–81.

6. Scott A, Docking S, Vicenzino B, et al. Sports and exercise-related tendinopathies: a review of selected topical issues by participants of the second International Scientific Tendinopathy Symposium (ISTS) Vancouver 2012. Br J Sports Med. 2013;47:536–44.

7. Copeland ST, Tipton JS, Fields KB. Evidence-based treatment of hamstring tears. Curr Sports Med Rep. 2009;8(6):308–14.

8. Wilson JJ, Best TM. Common overuse tendon problems: a review and recommendations for treatment. Am Fam Phys. 2005;72:811–8. (Internet) (Cited 2013 Jul 6). www.aafp.org/afp.

9. Carlson C. The natural history and management of hamstring injuries. Curr Rev Musculoskelet Med. 2008;1:120–3.

10. Sherry MA, Best TM. A comparison of 2 rehabilitation programs in the treatment of acute hamstring strains. J Orthop Sports Phys Ther. 2004;34(3):116–25.

11. Zebis MK, Skotte J, Andersen CH, et al. Kettlebell swing targets semitendinosus and supine leg curl targets biceps femoris: an EMG study with rehabilitation implications. Br J Sports Med. 2012. doi:10.1136/bjsports-2011-090281. (Published Online First).

12. Brukner P, Nealon A, Morgan C, et al. Recurrent hamstring muscle injury: applying the limited evidence in the professional football setting with a seven-point programme. Br J Sports Med. 2013. doi:10.1136/bjsports-2012-091400. (Published Online First).

13. Ahmad CS, Redler LH, Ciccotti MG, et al. Evaluation and management of hamstring injuries. Am J Sports Med. 2013;20(10):1–15. (Internet) (Cited 2013 Jul 6). http://www.sagepub.com/journalsPermissions.nav.

14. Cavalier R, Gabos PG, Bowen JR. Isolated rupture of the soleus muscle: a case report. Am J Orthop. 1998;27:755–7.

15. McClure JG. Gastrocnemius musculotendinous rupture: a condition confused with thrombophlebitis. South Med J. 1984;77:1143–5.

16. Dixon B. Gastrocnemius vs. soleus strain: how to differentiate and deal with calf muscle injuries. Curr Rev Musculoskelet Med. 2009;2:74–7.

17. Cardinal É, Rethy K. et al. Ultrasound-guided interventional procedures in the musculoskeletal system. Radiol Clin North Am. 1998;36(3):597–604.

18. Shields CL, Redix L, Brewster CE. Acute tears of the medial head of the gastrocnemius. Foot Ankle. 1985;5(4):186–90.

19. Kwak H-S, Han Y-M, Lee S-Y, et al. Diagnosis and follow-up US evaluation of ruptures of the medial head of the gastrocnemius ("tennis leg"). Korean J Radiol. 2006;7(3):193–8.

20. Elias DA, White LM, Rubenstein JD, et al. Clinical evaluation and MR imaging features of popliteal artery entrapment and cystic adventitial disease. Am J Roentgenol. 2003;180:627–32.

21. Tercan F, Oğuzkurt L, Kızılkılıç O, et al. Popliteal artery entrapment syndrome. Diagn Interv Radiol. 2005;11(4):222–4.

22. Nunes GS. Effect of Kinesio taping on jumping and balance in athletes: a cross-over randomized controlled trial. J Strength Cond Res. 2013;27:3183–9.

23. Stedge HL, Kroskie RM, Docherty CL. Kinesio taping and the circulation and endurance ratio of the gastrocnemius muscle. J Athl Train. 2012;47:635.

24. Perkins RH, Davis D. Musculoskeletal injuries in tennis. Phys Med Rehabil Clin N Am. 2006;17(3):609–631.

25. Touliopolous S, Hershman EB. Lower leg pain. Sports Med. 1999;27(3):193–204.

26. Campbell JT. Posterior calf injury. Foot Ankle Clin N Am. 2009;14(4):761–71.

27. Kwak HS, Lee KB, Han YM. Ruptures of the medial head of the gastrocnemius ("tennis leg"): clinical outcome and compression effect. Clin Imaging. 2006;30(1):48–53.

28. Nyland J, Lachman N, Kocabey Y, et al. Anatomy, function and rehabilitation of the popliteus musculotendinous complex. J Orthop Sports Phys Ther. 2005;35(3):165–179.

29. Blake SM, Treble NJ. Popliteus tendon tenosynovitis. Br J Sports Med. 2005;39:e42.

30. Hwang K, Lee KM, Han SH, Kim SG. Shape and innervation of popliteus muscle. Anat Cell Biol. 2012;43(2):165.

31. Hall CM, Brody LT. Therapeutic exercise moving toward function. 2nd ed. Philadelphia: Lippincott Williams and Wilkins; 2005. p. 283–308. Chapter 15, Closed kinetic chain training.

32. Fu SC, Hung LK, Shum WT, et al. In vivo low-intensity ultrasound following tendon injury promotes repair during granulation but suppresses dcorin and biglycan expression during remodeling. J Orthop Sports Phys Ther. 2010;40(7):422–9.

33. Pescasio M, Browning BB, Pedowitz RA. Clinical management of muscle strains and tears. J Musculoskelet Med. 2008;25(11):1–9.

34. Brown CL, Gilbert KK, Brismee JM, Sizer PS, James CR, Smith MP. The effects of neurodynamic mobilization on fluid dispersion within the tibial nerve at the ankle: an unembalmed cadaveric study. J Man Manip Ther. 2011;19(1):26–34.

35. Ellis RF, Hing WA, McNair PJ. Comparison of longitudinal sciatic nerve movement with different mobilization exercises: an in vivo study utilizing ultrasound imaging. J Orthop Sports Phys Ther. 2010;42(80):667–75.

36. Boyd BS, Topp KS, Coppieter MW. Impact of movement sequencing on sciatic and tibial nerve strain and excursion during the straight leg raise test in embalmed cadavers. J Orthop Sports Phys Ther. 2013;43(6):398–403.

37. Settergren R. Conservative management of a saphenous nerve entrapment in a female ultra-marathon runner. J Bodyw Mov Ther. 2013;17:297–301.

38. Howitt S, Jung S, Hammonds N. Conservative treatment of a tibialis posterior strain in a novice triathlete: a case report. J Can Chiropr Assoc. 2009;53(1):23–31.

39. Galbraith R, Lavallee ME. Medial tibial stress syndrome: conservative treatment options. Curr Rev Musculoskelet Med. 2009;2:127–33.

40. Kohls-Gatzoulis J, Angel JC, Singh D, Haddad F, Livingstone J, Berry G. Tibialis posterior dysfunction: a common and treatable cause of adult acquired flatfoot. Br Med J. 2004;329:1328–33.
41. Schon LC, DiStefano AF. Ecaluation and treatment of posterior tibialis tendinitis a case report and treatment protocol. J Dance Med Sci. 1999;3(1):24–7.
42. Wilson JJ, Best TM. Common overuse tendon problems: a review and recommendations for treatment. Am Fam Physician. 2005;72(5):811–8. (Review).
43. Jarvinen TA, Jarvinen TL, Kaariainen M, et al. Muscle injuries: optimizing recovery. Best Pract Res Clin Rheumatol. 2007;21:317–31. doi:10.1016/j.berh.2006.12.004.
44. Ferber R, a H, Kendall KD. Suspected mechanisms in the cause of overuse running injuries: a clinical review. Sports. 2009;1(3):242–6.
45. Beiner JM, Jokl P, Cholewicki J, et al. The effect of anabolic steroids and corcitosteroids on healing of muscle contusion injury. Am J Sports Med. 1999;27(1):2–9.
46. Markert CD, Merrick MA, Kirby TE, et al. Nonthermal ultrasound and exercise in skeletal muscle regeneration. Arch Phys Med Rehabil. 2005;86(7):1304–10.
47. Proske U, Morgan DL. Muscle damage from eccentric exercise: mechanism, mechanical signs, adaptation and clinical applications. J Physiol. 2001;537(Pt 2):333–45. (Review).
48. Michael R, Simpson, DO, MS, Thomas M, Howard, MD. Tendinopathies of the foot and ankle. Am Fam Physician. 2009;80(10):1107–14.
49. Doan-Johnson S. Flexor hallucis longus tenosynovitis. OrthopOne. 2012. http://www.orthopaedicsone.com/display/Main/Flexor+hallicus+longus+tenosynovitis.
50. George J, Kolettis MD, Lyle J, et al. Release of the Flexor hallucis longus tendon in ballet dancers. J Bone Joint Surg. 1996;78-A(9):1386–90.
51. Itzhak Siev-Ner MD. Common overuse Injuries of the foot and ankle in Dancers. J Dance Med Sci. 2000;4(2):49–53.
52. Christine L, Berglung SPT, Laura E, Philipps SPT, Sheyi Ojofeitimi MPT. Flexor hallucis longus tendinitis among dancers. Orthop Pract. 2006;18(3):26–31.
53. Conti SF, Wong YS. Foot and ankle injuries in the dancer. J Dance Med Sci. 2001;5(2):48.
54. Rowdon GA. Chronic exertional compartment syndrome. Updated Mar 7, 2013. http://emedicine.medscape.com/article/88014-overview.
55. American Academy of Orthopaedic Surgeons. Compartment syndrome. Last reviewed Oct. 2009. http://orthoinfo.aaos.org/topic.cfm?topic=A00204.
56. Varelas FL, Wessel J, Clement DB, Doyle DL, Wiley JP. Muscle function in chronic compartment syndrome of the leg. J Orthop Sports Phys Ther. 1993;18(5):586–589.
57. Forefoot Running for Chronic Exertional Compartment Syndrome. Posted on 30 May, 2012 by the sports physiotherapist in article review, blog, exercise prescription, foot and ankle, rehabilitation, sports physiotherapy, treatment. http://www.thesportsphysiotherapist.com/forefoot-running-for-chronic-exertional-compartment-syndrome/.
58. Knobloch, Karsten JM, et al. Eccentric training decreases paratendon capillary blood flow and preserves paratendon oxygen saturation in chronic Achilles tendinopathy. J Orthop Sports Phys Ther. 2007;37(5):269.
59. Sandmeier R, Renström PA. Diagnosis and treatment of chronic tendon disorders in sports. Scand J Med Sci Sports. 1997;7(2):96–106.
60. Neeter C, et al. Iontophoresis with or without dexamethazone in the treatment of acute Achilles tendon pain. Scand J Med Sci Sports. 2003;13(6):376–82.
61. Stanish WD, Mitchell Rubinovich R, Curwin S. Eccentric exercise in chronic tendinitis. Clin Orthop Relat Res. 1986;208:65–8.
62. Alfredson H, et al. Heavy-load eccentric calf muscle training for the treatment of chronic Achilles tendinosis. Am J Sports Med. 1998;26(3):360–6.
63. Miners AL, Bougie TL. Chronic Achilles tendinopathy: a case study of treatment incorporating active and passive tissue warm-up, Graston Technique®, ART®, eccentric exercise, and cryotherapy. J Can Chiropr Assoc. 2011;55(4):269.
64. Norregaard J, et al. Eccentric exercise in treatment of Achilles tendinopathy. Scand J Med Sci Sports. 2007;17(2):133–8.
65. Roos EM, et al. Clinical improvement after 6 weeks of eccentric exercise in patients with mid-portion Achilles tendinopathy–a randomized trial with 1-year follow-up. Scand J Med Sci Sports. 2004;14(5):286–95.
66. Wasielewski NJ, Kotsko KM. Does eccentric exercise reduce pain and improve strength in physically active adults with symptomatic lower extremity tendinosis? A systematic review. J Athl Train. 2007;42(3):409.
67. Sharma P, Maffulli N. Biology of tendon injury: healing, modeling and remodeling. J Musculoskelet Neuronal Interact. 2006;6(2):181.
68. Melham TJ, et al. Chronic ankle pain and fibrosis successfully treated with a new noninvasive augmented soft tissue mobilization technique (ASTM): a case report. Med Sci Sports Exerc. 1998;30:801–4.
69. McCormack JR. The management of mid-portion achilles tendinopathy with Astym® and eccentric exercise: a case report. Int J Sports Phys Ther. 2012;7(6):672.
70. Van Dijk CN, et al. Terminology for achilles tendon related disorders. Knee Surg Sports Traumatol Arthrosc. 2011;19(5):835–41.
71. Thomas JL, et al. The diagnosis and treatment of heel pain: a clinical practice guideline—revision 2010. J Foot Ankle Surg. 2010;49(3):S1–S19.
72. McBryde J, Angus M, Fred W, Ortmann IV. Retrocalcaneal bursoscopy. Tech Foot Ankle Surg. 2005;4(3):174–9.
73. Solan M, Davies M. Management of insertional tendinopathy of the Achilles tendon. Foot Ankle Clin N Am. 2007;12(4):597–615.
74. Yeung EW, Yeung SS. A systematic review of interventions to prevent lower limb soft tissue running injuries. Br J Sports Med. 2001;35(6):383–9.
75. Schepsis AA, Jones H, Haas AL. Achilles tendon disorders in athletes. Am J Sports Med. 2002;30(2):287–305.

76. Luk P, Thordarson D, Charlton T. Evaluation and management of posterior ankle pain in dancers. J Dance Med Sci. 2013;17(2):79–83.

77. Sofka CM. Posterior ankle Impingement: clarification and confirmation of the pathoanatomy. HSSJ. 2010;6:99–101.

78. Gasparetto F, Collo G, Pisanu G, Villella D, Drocco L, Cerlon R, Bonasia E. Posterior ankle and subtalar arthroscopy: indications, technique, and results. Curr Rev Musculoskelet Med. 2012;5:164–70.

79. Kadel NJ. Foot and ankle injuries in dance. Phys Med Rehabil Clin N Am. 2006;17:813–26.

80. DeLee JC, Drez's DD. Orthopaedic sports medicine. 3rd ed. Philadelphia: Saunders; 2009.

81. Howard PD. Differential diagnosis of calf pain and weakness: flexor hallucis longus strain. J Orthop Sports Phys Ther. 2000;30(2):78–84.

82. Cipriani DJ, Swartz JD, Hodgson CM. Triathlon and the multisport athlete. J Orthop Sports Phys Ther. 1998;27(2):42–50.

83. Albisetti W, Ometti M, Pascale V, De Bartolomeo O. Clinical evaluation and treatment of posterior impingement in dancers. Am J Phys Med Rehabil. 2009;88(5):349–54.

84. Smith TR. Management of dancers with symptomatic accessory navicular: 2 case reports. J Orthop Sports Phys Ther. 2012;42(5):465–73.

85. Vasukutty NV, Akrawi H, Theruvil B, Uglow M. Ankle arthroscopy in children. Ann R Coll Surg Engl. 2011;93:232–5.

86. Kolettis GJ, Micheli LJ, Klein JD. Release of the flexor hallucis longus tendon in ballet dancers. J Bone Joint Surg. 1996;78-A(9):1386–90.

87. Pommering TL, Kluchurosky L, Hall S. Ankle and foot injuries in pediatric and adult athletes. Prim Care Clin Office Pract. 2005;32:133–1.

88. Gillespie H. Osteochondroses and apophyseal injuries of the foot in the young athlete. Curr Sports Med Rep. 2010;9(5):265–68.

89. Cassas KJ, Cassettari-Wayhs A. Childhood and adolescent sport-related overuse injuries. Am Fam Physician. 2006;73:1014–22.

90. Cipriani DJ, Swartz JD, Hodgson CM. Triathlon and the multisport athlete. J Orthop Sports Phys Ther. 1998;27(1):42–50.

91. Howard PD. Differential diagnosis of calf pain and weakness: flexor hallucis longus strain. J Orthop Sports Phys Ther. 2000;30(2):78–84.

Special Population Considerations in the Treatment of Posterior Leg Injuries

Ryan R. Woods and Jeffrey S. Brault

Introduction

This chapter will provide an overview of possible risk factors for muscular injury, along with special considerations outside of the normal muscular injury diagnoses regarding lower limb musculature within the populations of pediatrics, female gender, the aging senior, and the previously injured/disabled. The mentioned populations each have their own variable intrinsic or extrinsic factors that may subject them to injury to the posterior lower limb; however, the biggest risk factor common to muscular injury is previous muscle injury. Previous muscle injury, in conjugation with insufficient rehabilitation, predisposes patients and athletes to reinjury within the same region [1]. This predisposition may be due in part to altered mechanical characteristics of the damaged muscle following injury [2]. Therefore, it is important that clinicians are not only aware of previous musculoskeletal injuries within their patient populations but also provide adequate treatment and rehabilitation. It is also vital for physicians to educate and stress the importance of prevention and tailor management to individual injuries, patient limitations, and patient goals.

Pediatric Population

Musculoskeletal system injuries within the pediatric population can provide a unique challenge to clinicians because of the many changes that take place during the developmental years.

Growth and Development The changes that take place in adolescents during the development, affect the muscles, bones, tendons, and ligaments in ways that predispose the pediatric population to injuries less commonly seen in adults. Tendons and ligaments are relatively stronger and more elastic compared to the epiphyseal plates; therefore, growth plate damage is more common in this group [3]. Those changes, along with structural abnormalities related to genetic or birth defects, can also predispose to injuries to the musculoskeletal system.

During the growth period, muscle growth lags behind bone growth. The gastrocnemius muscle displays one of the most functional examples of injury due to muscle growth lag [4]. The gastrocnemius, soleus, and plantaris muscles are the calf muscles that all conjoin and form the Achilles tendon, which inserts in the calcaneal apophysis. Given a child's imbalance of bone growth to muscle growth, the pediatric population is set up for increased muscle tension in the lower limbs due to structural changes during development. Increased muscle tightness of the gastrocnemius–soleus complex may therefore predispose adolescents to both muscle and tendon strains, along with other injuries, during

R. R. Woods (✉) · J. S. Brault
Department of Physical Medicine and Rehabilitation,
Mayo Clinic, Rochester, MN, USA
e-mail: Woods.Ryan@mayo.edu

J. S. Brault
e-mail: Brault.Jeffrey@mayo.edu

continual muscle activity [5]. This may also increase a child's risk for a certain apophysitis called Sever's disease [6]. Sever's disease is not directly related to injury of the calf muscle; however, the calf muscles play a role in the disease process through a traction apophysitis. Sever's disease typically affects children aged 9–11 years. The patient's presenting symptoms are usually bilateral heel pain while running or toe walking [7]. Sever's disease is very similar to Osgood–Schlatter disease in which repeated microtrauma leads to partial avulsion of the tendon insertion at the developing apophysis. Due to the normally dense and fragmented calcaneal apophysis normally found in many children, radiographs are usually not helpful in the diagnosis. Treatment includes nonsteroidal anti-inflammatory drugs (NSAIDs), padding of the heel, discontinuing wearing shoes contributing to damage, stretching the heel cord, and rest [7].

Also, during rapid growth, a tight gastrocnemius–soleus complex may cause a decrease in dorsiflexion in an adolescent patient. This decreased movement may change the biomechanics of the lower limb during function, for which surrounding structures must compensate. This alteration can, in turn, present increased risk of excessive foot pronation (flat foot), anterior ankle pain (impingement), and medial foot pain (plantar fasciitis) [4]. Anatomic or structural differences have been theorized to contribute to overuse injuries. Common conditions like pes cavus, pes planus, and calcaneal valgus may play a role in some injuries [3]. There are conflicting data about whether or not structural differences within the lower extremity lead to increased soft tissue injury. For example, a recent study demonstrated that muscle function of the gastrocnemius–soleus complex differed between individuals with low- and high-arched feet. Results reflected that the soleus muscle in a proportion of the subjects with low-arched feet showed a pattern of working harder during the forefoot loading phase when compared to subjects with high-arched feet [8]. These results only demonstrated trends, as no significant differences could be assessed between the two groups; nevertheless, this may show evidence that structural variation may

play a role in muscle function and injury. Conversely, studies have demonstrated no increased risk of lower limb overuse injury with pes planus or limb length inequalities [9, 10]. It is clear that further longitudinal studies sampling a variety of populations need to be done to assess better the issues of calf injury related to lower limb structural abnormalities.

Compartment Syndrome Chronic compartment syndrome has also been shown to occur in young athletes due to muscle hypertrophy and is commonly seen while running [3]. Pain, numbness, and tingling, associated with athletic activity, are often the presenting symptoms. Compartment syndrome can be both acute and chronic with acute development raising the potential of a medical emergency.

Growing Pains Pain in the lower limbs of a growing child can be a common complaint with a multitude of etiologies. A very common diagnosis, yet one of exclusion, for lower limb pain in children is growing pains. Growing pains usually begin in children aged 4–12 years [11, 12] and are described as bilateral musculoskeletal pains affecting the lower limbs, primarily the calf and thigh muscles. The etiology of growing pains is not known, and although they occur in growing children, they are not caused by growth. Pains do not occur at the sites of growth, do not affect the growth of children, and do not overlap with periods of growth [11]. Parents have commented on increasing episodes of pain after periods of increased physical activity. Other etiologies including fatigue, postural abnormalities related to orthopedic abnormalities, overuse, and restless leg syndrome have been proposed. Pains are described as crampy or restless in legs of older children aged 6–12 years [11]. Pains usually occur during the evenings and may interrupt sleep, being severe enough to induce crying in young children. Symptom-free periods range from days to months. Pains are generally relieved by massage, heat, or analgesics such as acetaminophen or ibuprofen. The pains do not alter normal activity or movement and are not specifically linked to joints. The differential diagnosis for pains in the lower extremity is extensive; it is important to rule out all other possibilities before designating calf and thigh pain as growing pains. Serious conditions that must be ruled out when considering a diagnosis of growing pains include but are not limited to trauma, tumor, infection, osteonecrosis, and vascular pathology [11]. The natural history of growing pains is a benign one. The pain is treated symptomatically and will subside eventually within a year or two of onset as the child matures [11]. If symptoms progress to a point that they affect movement or activity, or involve worsening pain, pain during the day or activity, or if the child becomes ill, it is important to get a full workup to either exclude or diagnose a more serious cause of the pain.

Viral Myositis Relative to other populations, the pediatric population can be more susceptible to viral myositis. There have been cases of myositis during outbreaks of influenza A and B [7]. Viral myositis is a benign, self-limiting illness that presents with muscle pain, tenderness, and sometimes swelling. The calf muscles of the lower limb are most commonly affected. Children will present with refusal to walk on their toes, and their calf muscles will be tender to palpation. It is possible for muscle enzyme to elevate up to 20–30 times the normal; however, myoglobinuria and acute renal failure have not been reported [7]. Muscle biopsy is not needed to diagnose viral myositis, but it does reveal evidence of muscle necrosis and muscle fiber regeneration. As stated previously, viral myositis is self-limiting, and recovery is seen in 3–10 days with resolution of the elevated muscle enzymes within 3 weeks [7].

Neuropathy/Myopathy

Cerebral Palsy Cerebral palsy (CP) is a neurological disorder causing lesions of the brain during development that can lead to impairments of the neurological and musculoskeletal system, usually manifesting as spasticity, dystonia, muscle contractures, bony deformities, incoordination, and muscle weakness [13]. Spastic muscles undergo significant changes during development,

often undergoing shortening to create muscle contractures, leading to joint contractures, decreased range of motion (ROM), and increased tone and stiffness [14, 15]. This sequence can lead to loss of function of the affected skeletal muscles and limb movement with declining functional ability over time. The lower limbs of children with CP and the muscles responsible for locomotion are often affected.

There have been conflicting reports regarding the physiological and structural changes within the affected skeletal muscle of CP patients. A commonly cited study conducted by Malaiya et al. showed the medial gastrocnemius of CP children aged 4–12 years to have a reduced physiological cross-sectional area, but no significant difference in fascicle length when compared to typically developed matched children [16]. This study took into account muscle volume, fascicle length, and pennation angle. A more recent study used ultrasound to study skeletal muscle in children aged 2–5 years with hemiplegic and diplegic spastic CP [14]. The results reflect medial gastrocnemius muscle volumes were 22% less in the group with spastic CP than in the typically developed group. Results reflected a significant difference between volumes, but no significant differences in fascicle length or pennation angle at a neutral ankle angle. However, changes were seen with plantar flexion in the later measures [14].

The study theorized that the change in muscle volume and physiological cross-sectional area (PCSA) were due to a reduced number of muscle fibers in parallel and decreased muscle fiber in a cross-sectional area [14]. Spastic muscles in children with CP have also been shown to have altered fiber sizes and fiber type distributions [15]. This may also contribute to the varying muscle volumes seen in CP patients.

Conversely, studies using magnetic resonance imaging (MRI) and ultrasound to assess lower limb muscles in children affected by CP demonstrated a decrease in mean muscle volume of six major lower limb muscles as a whole (by 18%) in CP patients. In spite of this, there was no significant difference in muscle volumes of the gastrocnemius and soleus specifically. However, in these studies the gastrocnemius muscle length was significantly reduced in CP patients. There was also evidence that suggested the Achilles tendon of patients with CP was longer, with a smaller cross-sectional area [13, 15].

Regardless, these studies suggest children with CP display muscle growth alterations that can decrease the volume and length of the gastrocnemius muscles; this, in turn, reduces the maximal muscle force production of the affected limbs and muscles and contributes to the functional limitations that these children display. Recent studies have demonstrated that muscle properties of children with CP may be altered at the cellular level [15]. Therefore, both structural and cellular alterations may affect the mechanical performance of skeletal muscles in children with CP. It is important for clinicians to be aware of these structural changes to better assess and treat patients affected by CP.

There will be a need for longitudinal studies of the natural history of muscle growth during development of CP patients, taking into account the extent of the brain lesions, the degree of motor impairment, and the level of functioning in relation to muscle structure properties in spastic CP patients [14].

Duchenne Muscular Dystrophy Duchenne muscular dystrophy (DMD) is a fatal, X-linked muscle-wasting disease seen in male patients caused by the absence of the membrane-associated cytoskeletal protein *dystrophin,* due to mutation of the dystrophin gene. DMD is characterized by the progressive loss of contractile function, muscle weakness, and progressive degeneration of muscle tissue with replacement by noncontractile fat and connective tissue [17]. DMD onset is usually around 3–5 years and usually presents with intellectual impairment, in addition to speech and motor delays. Fast-twitch fibers are particularly susceptible to myopathy with DMD [18]. The muscle involvement is bilateral and symmetrical and normally affects the lower limbs first. A common finding is pseudohypertrophy of the gastrocnemii, in which they appear to be larger than normal but exhibit progressive muscle weakness [17]. DMD generally affects the proximal muscles more than the distal ones; however,

the gastrocnemii are normally involved. Affected muscles are more prone to injuries occurring with repeated strain, including repeated lengthening, or eccentric contractions of sufficient load and frequency to induce fatigue injury in skeletal muscles. The load magnitude required to induce muscle damage with repeated eccentric contractions in DMD patients is much lower than that of typical normal muscles [18]. The absence of dystrophin renders muscle cells more vulnerable to damage by mechanical stress, possibly through a more injury-susceptible sarcolemma [17]. Along with increased susceptibility to injury, muscle repair in DMD patients is ineffective. One theory is that multiple rounds of degeneration and regeneration deplete the satellite cell pool responsible for muscle regeneration [17]. Therefore, patients diagnosed with DMD are at higher risk for muscle injury and damage than the general population, including distally affected muscles such as the gastrocnemii. Clinicians should be aware of the possibility of DMD in pediatric patients who present with calf complaints, including bilateral hypertrophy associated with delays or difficulty in ambulation.

Idiopathic Toe Walking

Idiopathic toe walking (ITW) is a gait abnormality illustrated by persistent toe walking without a normal heel-to-toe pattern, caused by an unspecific etiology. Toe walking is part of developmental ambulation and considered fairly normal in children, less than 2 years of age, learning to walk. Continued toe walking beyond the age of 2 years, however, warrants further investigation, as toe walking can be an early sign of a developmental disorder [19].

Toe walking usually presents bilaterally, and after 2 years of age is considered idiopathic if there is no discernible cause. Possible etiologies of ITW have been hypothesized to be due to structural differences within the Achilles tendon or difference within the fiber type of the gastrocnemius; however, the etiology remains largely unknown [19]. There are limited data surrounding the natural history of ITW. Studies show various outcomes, including both the improvement of gait to normal heel-to-toe pattern, along with other cases showing no improvement. Management includes nonoperative treatments, including physical therapy along with bracing, splinting, casting, and stretching. Surgical treatments include lengthening of the triceps surae group via percutaneous Achilles tendon lengthening, or invasive lengthening of the gastrocnemius muscle itself [19].

Observation for children less than 2 years of age who are learning to walk is the best initial treatment for toe walking. However, clinicians must be aware of possible etiologies and conditions associated with toe walking, which must be investigated further if toe walking persists, worsens, or becomes associated with other symptoms during child development.

Female Population

Gender roles affecting the musculoskeletal system have been a topic of interest. Hormones, in addition to contributing sexual characteristics and function in females, have been shown to play a role in many other tissues and organs. Of interest to the scope of this chapter, estrogen has been shown to have effects on skeletal muscles, possibly providing for a difference in gender regarding the regulation and function of the musculoskeletal system.

Hormonal Influence Estrogen has been shown to influence many aspects of muscle physiology and function, along with potentially influencing muscle damage, inflammation, and repair [20]. There have been a number of mechanisms thought responsible for the ability of estrogen to have such an influence, including antioxidant properties, possible membrane stabilization, and inhibition of neutrophil and leukocyte infiltration during the post-damage inflammatory response [20].

A number of animal studies have demonstrated the possible protective effect of estrogen on skeletal muscles, specifically the gastrocnemius muscle in rats undergoing acute muscle strain in-

jury. One particular study used plasma creatine kinase (CK) as a marker of muscle damage, and compared the levels of CK in different groups of female mice that were ovariectomized and exogenously treated with variable dosages of estradiol. The results reflected a decreased rise in serum CK after muscle strain in the rats with intact ovaries and ones receiving estrogen administration. The study also followed indices for antioxidants and muscle regeneration. Researchers concluded that estrogen provided protection from primary stretch injury, possibly through membrane stabilization, and from secondary muscle damage through antioxidation [21].

Hormonal Imbalances It has been shown that female athletes with sports-induced amenorrhea or oligomenorrhea have decreased serum levels of estradiol [22]. Therefore, this population of females may not benefit from the protective influence that estrogen may have on skeletal muscles, thereby increasing their risk for muscle damage and impaired muscle regeneration.

Similarly, postmenopausal females, who are not on hormone replacement therapy (HRT), have decreased levels of serum estrogens. It is possible that this population would also not benefit from estrogen influence on muscle damage and repair and be at an increased risk for injury. An animal study [23] tested the effects of estrogen administration on immobilization-induced soleus muscle atrophy in male rats. Researchers found that compared to the placebo group, estrogen treatment significantly reduced muscle atrophy by 35% after 10 days of immobilization.

HRT is widely known and used to protect females against osteoporosis. Studies raise the question of the protective effect that estrogen has on the muscle and if estrogen therapy may have a role in age-related muscle atrophy in the postmenopausal population. A double-blind study tested this theory on women aged 50–57 [24]. The subjects were randomly assigned to groups that consisted of exercise alone, HRT, HRT + exercise, and a control group. Among their measured outcomes were lean tissue cross-sectional areas of the quadriceps and lower leg muscles. The results of the study showed a significant increase in lean cross-sectional area of the quadriceps and lower leg muscles in the HRT group when compared to the control. The exercise alone and the HRT + exercise also showed increases in lean tissue mass of the quadriceps and lower leg muscles, with the HRT + exercise group having the highest increase of all the groups [24]. This study demonstrated that HRT has an influence on muscle mass. The results support the notion that estrogens play a beneficial role in muscle maintenance. However, further studies are needed to define a mechanism and clinical significance for the possible protective effect estrogen has on muscle atrophy.

Gender Kinematics Gender differences not only include hormonal differences, but also structural and possible kinematic differences. For example, it has been well documented that female athletes are at increased risk for anterior cruciate ligament (ACL) injury compared to their male counterparts. A recent study set out to find differences involving kinematics as a possible contributing factor to increased ACL injuries in female athletes [25]. The study demonstrated a surprising difference in gastrocnemius muscle activity in female soccer players compared to their male counterparts during specific maneuvers. Female subjects demonstrated greater activation of lateral and medial gastrocnemius activity compared to the males; furthermore, researchers found that the female athletes had a mediolateral muscle imbalance, with the lateral gastrocnemius being more active than the medial gastrocnemius. This was one of the first studies to demonstrate a gender difference in muscle activity and an imbalance within the gastrocnemius of females during specific maneuvers [25]. Although the target of this study was to identify risk factors for ACL injury, it may have provided evidence for kinematic differences between males and females regarding muscle function that may influence the risk of muscle strain or overuse injuries. Further studies are warranted to investigate the possibility of different kinematics and the clinical significance they may have. However, clinicians should be aware of possible differences when assessing and treating females for activity-induced injury.

Pregnancy Many changes across many organ systems take place during pregnancy. Of interest to the scope of this chapter are the possible effects that take place within the lower limb musculature.

Many conditions, as well as medications, can predispose to cramping. Cramps are not specific to any gender or population; however, pregnant women have been shown to have a somewhat increased frequency of cramping compared to the general population, especially during the later months [26, 27]. Cramps are painful, involuntary contractions of skeletal muscles, normally affecting the muscles of the lower limb, specifically the calf muscles. They can affect people of any age and gender and occur at any time of the day. Muscle cramping typically has a sudden onset with resolution within 10 min.

Clinicians should be mindful that pregnant woman may be more prone to muscle cramping and provide education, therapy, and possible prevention through nondrug interventions such as stretching, massage, exercise, changes in footwear, and reassurance [27]. There are also medications to treat severe cramping; however, any drug therapies should be discussed with the patient's obstetrician/gynecologist (OB/GYN), as certain medications may pose a risk to the pregnancy.

Disuse atrophy is a common concept surrounding muscular function. Research shows that bed rest induces many physiologic changes, including changes to the musculoskeletal system [28]. Muscles of the lower limb are most susceptible to bed rest-induced disuse atrophy. A study set out to investigate the effects of bed rest on the gastrocnemius muscle of pregnant woman. Results reflected that woman put on antepartum bed rest for a mean of 24.8 days underwent changes in muscle metabolism measured by muscle tissue oxygenation and deoxygenation. It was determined that the length of time for the gastrocnemius muscle to reoxygenate after exercise correlated with muscle deconditioning. They found that reoxygenation time significantly increased from the time the patient was admitted and put on bed rest until discharge. Patients were followed for 6 weeks postpartum. Patients also self-reported symptoms of muscle decondition-ing that included leg muscle soreness, fatigue, cramping, and muscle tears [28]. The research-ers found that reoxygenation time decreased dur-ing the 6 weeks postpartum following exercise, demonstrating the belief that muscle atrophy occurs during antepartum bed rest and recovers during the postpartum and remobilization [28]. It is important for clinicians to be aware that bed rest patients—including, but not limited to preg-nant patients—may be prone to muscle injury upon ambulation and weight-bearing following a prolonged bed rest. Specifically at risk are the lower limb muscles in charge of postural control and ambulation. Postpartum physical therapy targeting the lower limb, specifically the gastroc-nemius and soleus, may provide prevention of injury and aid in a quicker recovery of strength, balance, and mobility.

Aging/Senior Population

The aging population today is not only living longer but also staying active longer as well. The increase in the aging population, along with the interest in continued physical function and exer-cise, is resulting in increasing risk of musculo-skeletal injuries to the senior population.

Aging-Related Muscle Effects Aging affects the body across many systems. The purpose of this section is to provide an overview of the effects aging has on muscle, injury, and frailty within the aging population. It is well known that aging causes a decrease in muscle mass and muscle strength, therefore, decreasing muscle function. *Sarcopenia* is the term used to describe muscular changes occurring during the aging process. Sar-copenia leads to an increase in physical frailty, affecting mobility and increasing risk for falls and other musculoskeletal injuries. Peak perfor-mance and muscle mass start to decline during the third decade of life, with an average loss of 15% of muscle mass between the ages of 30 and 60 and an average loss of 30% after the age of 60 [29]. Both the decrease in total muscle fibers and the decrease in the cross-sectional area of the

remaining fibers contribute to the loss of muscle mass in the aging population [30]. These losses in muscle fiber number and mass decrease both strength and stamina as one ages. Interestingly, studies show that type two muscle fibers are dis-proportionally decreased when compared to type one muscle fibers [29]. Literature seems to show conflicting data regarding the changes made to muscle fibril length and pennation angle in the aging process; however, it is clear that muscular function declines with age.

Muscle injury occurs most frequently with lengthening or eccentric contractions. Ultrasound evidence has shown mechanical damage within and between sarcomeres during contraction-in-duced muscle injury [30]. Animal studies have shown evidence suggesting that muscles of older rats are more susceptible to injury than those of younger rats, partly because aged sarcomeres are mechanically compromised relative to younger muscle, and therefore not as able to withstand stretch [30]. This idea of increased injury sus-ceptibility due to stretch describes the potential mechanical difference in contractile proteins between young and old, therefore increasing the risk of injury in the aging population. Other stud-ies regarding sarcomere function have hypoth-esized that there is an increase in the number of weak sarcomeres in series of myofibrils. This imbalance of sarcomeres may result in increased risk of injury during stretch and would again suggest that aged muscles are more susceptible to damage [30]. Recovery from injury has also been shown to be an issue affecting the muscles of both older animals and humans alike. This should also be taken into consideration follow-ing the acute injury and rehabilitation of a senior patient. Animal studies have suggested that the environment surrounding aging muscle lacks or has decreased factors important to the regenera-tion of muscle, possibly involving the activation satellite cells [30].

Regarding the gastrocnemius specifically, studies have shown both a decrease in muscle force and muscle cross-sectional area of the lat-eral head of the gastrocnemius in men with an average age of 73.8 years, compared to young men with an average age of 25.3 years [31].

The selective atrophy of type two fibers, along with decreased fiber tension, is thought to play the biggest role in the decreased muscle force production. The study demonstrated a greater loss in cross-sectional area than fascicle length, thereby suggesting the difference in volume between young and old muscles may be due to a decrease of sarcomeres in parallel rather than in series. The study also found that the pennation angle was 12 % smaller in elderly men. The study goes on to say that it is also likely that both increased intramuscular connective tissue and fat, along with denervated fibers, contribute to the decrease in muscle force production in the senior population [31]. Along with intrinsic muscle changes, the study also considered that reduced physical activity plays a role in reduced muscle mass and force. A different study comparing the muscle architecture showed no significant difference in pennation angle or relative (to limb length) muscle thickness of the medial gastrocnemius in young and elderly patients; however, a significantly smaller absolute muscle cross-sectional area was seen [32]. Interestingly, this study showed a greater loss in muscle thickness of the knee extensor muscles than the plantar flexors. This may be due in part to the higher activation level of the plantar flexors during normal locomotion, which may again show decreased physical activity being a component of age-related muscle changes.

Aging Biomechanical Effects on Muscle In addition to intrinsic muscle changes, biomechanical differences between young and old may contribute to injury. A recent study investigated the kinematics in runners aged 55–65 compared to younger runners of 20–35 [33]. Researchers used both self-selected and controlled speeds to assess. The study showed that the older group displayed a larger impact force and initial loading rate than the younger group. Results also showed at both speeds, the older study group demonstrated differences in knee flexion at heel strike along with differences in total knee flexion and extension ROM. The larger impact forces are thought to be due to the loss of shock-absorbing ability in the aged runners, due to the musculo-

skeletal degeneration of aging. It was also noted that the older runners had a significantly shorter stride than the younger runners, thereby allowing an increased frequency of repetitive forces on the lower extremities compared to their younger counterparts. It is possible that these changes in biomechanics and musculoskeletal properties make the elderly population more susceptible to overuse injuries within the lower extremity [33].

Injury Prevention Muscle decline with aging is evident. However, studies have shown that low-impact exercises and stretching, along with proper nutrition, can be beneficial to the age-related declines in muscle mass, strength, and function and increased susceptibility to injury. Studies have demonstrated that regular heel raise training not only improved muscle mass in the soleus and gastrocnemius in woman aged 60–79 years but also improved posture control and balance [34, 35]. Furthermore, this training was easy to perform within this population. Along with improvements in muscle secondary to weight-bearing exercise, passive stretching has been shown to be beneficial in the prevention of contraction-induced injuries [30]. Mice exposed to a conditioning protocol of passive stretching prior to undergoing a lengthening contraction protocol showed a decreased number of damaged fibers 3 days post contraction protocol compared to mice that did not undergo the conditioning protocol [30]. The passive stretching also proved to be non-damaging to the muscle; therefore, this study concluded that conditioning muscle with passive stretching exercises can be a safe and effective way to decrease the risk of injury within the aging population [30].

Additional Aging Changes Studies have shown that proper nutrition and hormone replacement may act as preventive/protective methods to maintain muscle health in the senior population. As estrogen has shown some protective muscular effects, studies have demonstrated that an increase of serum testosterone in elderly men correlated with the preservation of muscle thickness in the gastrocnemius at 6 months when compared to the placebo group, suggesting that there is a possible hormonal influence on the muscular aging process. The authors concluded that the effects of testosterone most likely halted or slowed the decrease in muscle architecture, but did not cause hypertrophy of the muscles themselves due to lack of major changes in the pennation angle and fascicle length of the muscle [36]. Nutrition has also been shown to affect muscle. Malnutrition has been correlated with lower muscle mass and strength, along with changes in metabolic properties of elderly patients [37]. Nutritional repletion could be a very easy corrective means to improve muscle function within the elderly population.

Calf Pain Muscle strain is one of the most common lower extremity injuries; furthermore, most muscle strain injuries involve the gastrocnemius–soleus complex. The majority of aging athletes who present with acute pain in the calf region suffer from a tear that involves the medial gastrocnemius. This injury is usually due to an eccentric contraction during dorsiflexion accompanied by knee extension, and has been termed *tennis leg*. Due to its biarticular structure and dominance of type two muscle fibers, the gastrocnemius is at greatest risk for this type of injury. In addition to common muscle strains, other injuries to consider in the aged patient presenting with lower leg/calf pain include: stress fractures, shin splints, compartment syndrome, arthritis, both a ruptured and unruptured Baker cyst, claudication secondary to peripheral vasculature disease, deep vein thrombosis, and drug-induced conditions including myopathy secondary to statin drug therapy and other interactions [29].

In conclusion, further studies are needed in order to better understand the mechanisms and results that aging has on the musculoskeletal system. The aging effects on the musculoskeletal system are largely irreversible; however, with a proper understanding of the changes taking place during the aging process, in combination with potential muscle-preserving techniques, clinicians may improve function with the elderly population, decrease injury risk, and help to maintain a higher quality of life within our ever-increasing aging population.

Disabled/Previously Injured

Spinal Injuries Injuries to the spinal cord have obvious detrimental effects to the musculoskeletal system. Lower extremity paresis and resultant muscle atrophy are debilitating complications following a complete spinal cord injury.

The study of incomplete spinal cord injury and its effects on the musculoskeletal system is not as well defined, even though this population accounts for 51 % [38] of new spinal cord injuries.

Researchers have studied the extent of lower extremity muscle atrophy following an incomplete spinal cord injury using MRI to compare the difference in muscle cross-sectional area between patients with incomplete spinal cord injury and age-, sex-, height-, and weight-matched controls [38]. Furthermore, researchers divided the injured patients into those who use a wheelchair for mobility and those who use other means of assisted mobility if needed. Not surprisingly, results revealed significant atrophy of the lower extremity muscles—mean loss of 24–31 % in the injured group compared to the controls—with greater atrophy of the posterior compartment of the lower leg when compared to the muscles of the thigh. The degree of muscle atrophy in the study patients with incomplete injuries compared to the reported atrophy of patients with complete spinal cord injuries was much less, almost half. It is thought that the partial preservation of motor control during incomplete spinal cord injury allows variable activation of spared muscle groups. Atrophy after a spinal cord injury occurs due to both the initial injury to the motor neurons and the subsequent inactivation of the innervated muscles.

This idea of variable activation of spared motor neurons and muscle atrophy was supported when the study divided the group into wheelchair and non-wheelchair users. It was found that the wheelchair-user group had greater atrophy of the plantar flexor muscles and showed a significantly greater amount of atrophy in the medial gastrocnemius, with no significant differences in the thigh musculature, when compared to the non-wheelchair group [38]. It was thought the greater amount of atrophy was due to the fact that weight-bearing and mechanical loading on the lower extremity of the wheelchair group was less, as the ability to walk would be more difficult compared to an individual who uses a different form of assistive device such as a walker or crutch. In addition, it was suggested that the flexed position of the knee for extended periods in the wheelchair group could have contributed to shortening of the gastrocnemius muscle, resulting in increased atrophy when compared to the non-wheelchair group [38].

This study demonstrates that an incomplete spinal cord injury will result in muscle atrophy of the affected segments with risk of the greatest atrophy in the musculature of the posterior lower limbs. Atrophy may also be variable, depending on the extent of injury and number of spared motor units, allowing for preservation of some weight bearing and mobility. Furthermore, these results may suggest that any individual walking with any assistive device allowing for decreased loading on the lower extremities may suffer from mild atrophy of the lower limb musculature. Direct injury to the spinal cord is not the only mechanism by which muscle atrophy of the lower limb can occur. Lumbosacral stenosis can cause radiculopathy that may present with multiple symptoms, one of which can be muscle atrophy of the nerve-root distribution [39]. During the treatment process it is important to at least consider the possibility of either present atrophy or future atrophy in the lower limb in a patient presenting with a lower lumbosacral radiculopathy.

Although much more rare than neurogenic muscular atrophy, muscle hypertrophy can be a complication of denervation. Interestingly, most neurogenic hypertrophies involve the calf muscles and, when occurring unilaterally, are usually caused by an S1 radiculopathy [39]. When occurring bilaterally, etiologies such as anterior horn cell disease or polyneuropathy can be considered. The majority of pathologic muscle hypertrophy is due to myopathic disorders; however, there are other causes, including inflammatory myopathies and muscle infiltration from such things as neoplasm that could be the etiology [39].

It is important for clinicians to be aware of the variability in muscle response due to changes in innervation, whether due to spinal cord injury, spinal stenosis, peripheral nerve injury, or stroke. Being aware of the possible causes and effects of given injuries and the muscle responses that follow will help clinicians provide better rehab strategies, thereby reducing the risk of subsequent musculoskeletal injuries.

Amputee Unilateral lower extremity amputees suffer from biomechanical variations during gait and may be predisposed to injury to their non-injured lower extremity. An article studying the soft tissue injuries to US Paralympians showed that athletes who used unilateral lower extremity prostheses suffered from an increase in ankle injuries compared to other populations [40]. This study also cited articles demonstrating differences in asymmetry and force production in the non-impaired lower extremities of amputee patients compared to normal controls. It would make sense that altered biomechanical properties of gait due to injury must be balanced by increased effort within remaining intact structures. A recent study looked into the co-contraction patterns of the ankle and knee musculature of transtibial amputees. Results reflected that compared to normal control groups, there was an increase in co-contraction levels of ankle musculature, including the medial gastrocnemius, within the intact limbs of amputees during the majority of the gait cycle. This mechanism was thought to be a compensatory strategy to provide additional stability and support during locomotion [41]. Prosthetic devices have come a long way and allow for an improved quality of life in many amputee patients; however, they are not biomechanically equal to the human ankle. Para athletes are becoming increasingly more active, and in doing so they are pushing their prostheses to perform at higher levels. Researchers have shown an increase in ankle injury during running when compared to walking. This suggests that there is a difference in force production and mechanics during variable gait speeds and that prosthetics set up for lower-energy motion may not be adequate for running or higher levels of activity, and therefore increase risk of injury [40]. Furthermore, technological advances in lower limb prosthetics will provide for an increase in energy-storing ability of the prosthesis, and could possibly increase the force that develops around the musculature and joint of the non-impaired leg that may predispose to further injury in the normal lower extremity [40].

Altered biomechanics and the increase in load and activity seen in the intact limb of amputees put this population at risk for additional muscular injuries. Clinicians must be aware of the importance of proper fitting and tailoring of prosthetics to patient-specific activities to help reduce the stress on the non-prosthetic lower extremity and help improve overuse injuries within this population.

Altered Biomechanics Overuse injuries due to gait are not only a concern within the amputee population. A recent study demonstrated that variable gait patterns within the general population can be a factor for lower limb overuse injuries. The study showed that patients who had less foot pronation during heel strike, along with a more lateral roll-off, were at increased risk for lower limb overuse injuries [42]. Alternatively, another proposed hypothesis for increased risk of overuse injury is excessive foot pronation; there is evidence to both support and reject foot pronation as a cause for increased lower limb injury [43]. The intrinsic factors contributing to these variable gait patterns and injury are unclear [42]. Nonetheless, it is important for physicians to be aware of the possible biomechanical issues affecting lower limb function and predisposition to injury. Clinicians should take the time to observe gait in their patients and provide any additional therapy to increase support and decrease stress within the musculature and joints surrounding the lower limb through taping or orthotics [44].

Conclusions

Muscular injury plagues people of all ages. This chapter highlights some of the specific issues concerning gastrocnemius muscle injury or dysfunction within the given populations of pediatrics, female gender, aging seniors, and the previously injured/disabled. Clinicians need to be aware of the intrinsic and extrinsic differences between their patients that may render them more

susceptible to injury or muscular issues outside the normal diagnoses. Much research still needs to be done to assess mechanisms for and clinical relevance of many topics previously covered within this chapter. Nonetheless, it is important for clinicians to be aware of differences across patient populations. A better understanding of possible etiologies and issues unique to individual patients and patient populations leads to better care and patient quality of life, which is something valued across all populations.

References

1. Murphy DF, Connolly DA, Beynnon BD. Risk factors for lower extremity injury: A review of the literature. www.bjsportmed.com (2002).
2. Garrett WE Jr. Muscle strain injuries. Am J Sports Med. 1996;24:S2–8.
3. Bruns W, Maffulli N. Lower limb injuries in children in sports. Clin Sports Med. 2000;19:637–62.
4. Grady MF, Goodman A. Common lower extremity injuries in the skeletally immature athletes. Curr Probl Pediatr Adolesc Health Care. 2010;40(7):170–83.
5. Brukner P, Khan K. Clinical sports medicine (4th ed.). North Ryde: McGraw-Hill; 2012.
6. Frank JB, Jarit GJ, Bravman JT, Rosen JE. Lower extremity injuries in the skeletally immature athlete. J Am Acad Orthop Surg. 2007;15:356–66.
7. Clark MC. Overview of the causes of limp in children. www.uptodate.com (2012).
8. Branthwaite H, Pandyan A, Chockalingam N. Function of the triceps surae muscle group in low and high arched feet: an exploratory study. Foot. 2012;22:56–9.
9. Michelson JD, Durant DM, McFarland E. The injury risk associated with pes planus in athletes. Foot Ankle Intl. 2002, July;23:629–33.
10. Gross DL, Moore JH, Slivka EM, Halter BS. Comparison of injury rates between cadets with limb length inequalities and matched control subjects over 1 year of military training and athletic participation. Mil Med. 2006;171:522–5.
11. Lehman TJ. Growing pains. www.uptodate.com. 2012.
12. Halliwell P, Monsell F. Growing pains: a diagnosis of exclusion. The Practitioner; 2001
13. Gao F, Zhao H, Gaebler-Spira D, Zhang L. In vivo evaluations of morphologic changes of gastrocnemius muscle fascicles and Achilles tendon in children with cerebral palsy. Am J Phys Med Rehabil. 2011;90:364–71.
14. Barber L, Hastings-Ison T, Baker R, Barrett R, Lichtwark G. Medial gastrocnemius muscle volume and fascicle length in children aged 2 to 5 years with cerebral palsy. Dev Med Child Neurol. 2011;53: 543–8.

15. Oberhofer K, Stott N, Mithraratne K, Anderson I. Subject-specific modeling of lower limb muscles in children with cerebral palsy. Clin Biomech. 2010;25:88–94.

16. Malaiya R, McNee AE, Fry NR, Eve LC, Gough M, Shortland AP. The morphology of the medial gastrocnemius in typically developing children and children with spastic hemiplegic cerebral palsy. J Electromyogr Kinesiol. 2007;17:657–63.

17. Gainer TG, Wang Q, Ward CW, Grange RW. Duchenne muscular dystrophy. In: Tiidus PM, editor. Skeletal muscle damage and repair. Champaign: Human Kinetics; 2008. pp. 113–23.

18. Lawler JM. Exacerbation of pathology by oxidative stress in respiratory and locomotor muscles with Duchenne muscular dystrophy. J Physiol. 2011;589(9): 2161–70.

19. Oetgen ME, Peden S. Idiopathic toe walking. J Am Acad Orthop Surg. 2012;20:292–300.

20. Tiidus PM. Estrogen and gender effects. In: Tiidus PM, editor. Skeletal muscle damage and repair. Champaign: Human Kinetics; 2008. pp. 125–34.

21. Feng X, LI G, Wang S. Effects of estrogen on gastrocnemius muscle strain injury and regeneration in female rats. Act Pharmacological Sonica. 2004;25:1489–94.

22. Salsa T, Airy K, Yoshida N, Ishikawa M, Fukunaga M. Effects of ovariectomy on intramuscular energy metabolism in young rats: how does sports-related-amenorrhea affect muscles of young female athletes. J Physiol Anthropol Appl Human Sci. 20(2):125–9.

23. Sugiura T, Ito N, Goto K, Naito H, Yoshioka T, Powers SK. Estrogen administration attenuates immobilization-induced skeletal muscle atrophy in male rats. J Physiol Sci. 2006;56:393–9.

24. Sipila S, Taaffe DR, Cheng S, Puolakka J, Toivanen J, Suominen H. Effects of hormone replacement therapy and high-impact physical exercise on skeletal muscle in post-menopausal women: a randomized placebo-controlled study. Clin Sci. 2001;101:147–57.

25. Landry SC, McKean KA, Hubley-Kozey CL, Stanish WD, Deluzio KJ. Neuromuscular and lower limb biomechanical differences exist between male and female elite adolescent soccer players during an unanticipated side-cut maneuver. Am J Sports Med. 2007;35:1888–900.

26. Cohen JA, Mowchun J, Grudem J. Peripheral nerve and muscle disease. New York: Oxford University Press; 2009.

27. Blyton F, Chuter V, Walter KE, Burns J. Non-drug therapies for lower limb muscle cramps. Cochrane Database Syst Rev. 2012;1:CD008496.

28. Maloni JA, Schneider BS. Inactivity: symptoms associated with gastrocnemius muscle disuse during pregnancy. AACN Clin Issues. 2002;13:248–62.

29. Prescott JW, Yu JS. The aging athlete: part I, "boomeritis" of the lower extremity. AJR. 2012;199:W294–306.

30. Brooks SV. Changes with aging. In: Tiidus PM, editor. Skeletal muscle damage and repair. Champaign: Human Kinetics; 2008. pp. 105–12.

31. Morse CI, Thom JM, Reeves ND, Birch KM, Narici MV. In vivo physiological cross-sectional area and specific force and reduced in the gastrocnemius of elderly men. J Appl Physiol. 2005;99:1050–5.

32. Kubo K, Kanehisa H, Azuma K, Ishizu M, Kuno S, Okada M, Fukunaga T. Muscle architectural characteristics in young and elderly men and women. Int J Sports Med. 2003;24:125–30.

33. Bus SA. Ground reaction forces and kinematics in distance running in older-aged men. Med Sci Sports Exerc. 2003;35(7):1167–75.

34. Fujiwara K, Toyama H, Asai H, Maeda K, Yaguchi C. Regular heel-raise training focused on the soleus for the elderly: evaluation of muscle thickness by ultrasound. J Physiol Anthropol. 2010;29(1):23–8.

35. Fujiwara K, Toyama H, Asai H, Yaguchi C, Irei M, Naka M, Kaida C. Effects of regular heel-raise training aimed at the soleus muscle on dynamic balance associated with arm movement in elderly women. J Strength Cond Res. 2011;25:2605–15.

36. Atkinson RA, Srinivas-Shankar U, Roberts SA, Connolly MJ, Adams JE, Oldham JA, Narici MV. Effects of testosterone on skeletal muscle architecture in intermediate-frail and frail elderly men. J Gerontol. 2010;65(11):1215–9.

37. Bourdel-Marchasson I, Joseph P, Dehail P, Biran M, Faux P, Rainfray M, Thiaudiere E. Functional and metabolic early changes in calf muscle occurring during nutritional repletion in malnourished elderly patients. Am J Clin Nutr. 2001;73:832–8.

38. Shah PK, Stevens JE, Gregory CM, Pathare NC, Jayaraman A, Bickel S, Vandenborne K. Lower-extremity muscle cross-sectional area after incomplete spinal cord injury. Arch Phys Med Rehabil. 2006;87:772–8.

39. Swartz KR, Fee DB, Trost GR, Waclawik AJ. Unilateral calf hypertrophy seen in lumbosacral stenosis. Spine. 2002;27:E406–9.

40. Nyland J, Snouse SL, Anderson M, Kelly T, Sterling JC. Soft tissue injuries to USA paralympians at the 1996 summer games. Arch Phys Med Rehabil. 2000;81:368–73.

41. Seyedali M, Czerniecki JM, Morgenroth DC, Hahn ME. Co-contraction patterns of trans-tibial amputee ankle and knee musculature during gait. J NeuroEng Rehabil. 2012;9(29):1–9.

42. Ghani Zadeh Hesar N, Van Ginckel A, Cools A, Peersman W, Roosen R, De Clercq D, Witvrouw E. A prospective study on gait-related intrinsic risk factors for lower leg overuse injuries. J Sports Med. 2009;43:1057–61.

43. Chuter VH, Janse de Jonge XA. Proximal and distal contributions to lower extremity injury: a review of the literature. Gait Posture. 2012;36:7–15.

44. Vicenzino B, Griffiths SR, Griffiths LA, Hadley A. Effect of antipronation tape and temporary orthotic on vertical navicular height before and after exercise. J Orthop Sports Phys Ther. 2000;30:333–9.

Complementary Medicine Practices for Muscular Injuries of the Posterior Leg

Bo M. Rowan[†] and J. Bryan Dixon

Introduction

Complementary treatments for musculoskeletal injuries commonly include manual therapies such as traditional Chinese medicine (TCM), osteopathic manipulation, chiropractic medicine, naprapathic medicine, massage therapy, injection therapies, and transdermal modalities. Many of these treatments have been used for years, in some cases thousands of years, as an alternative to standard treatments. However, the evidence for these modalities is often only anecdotal at best due to lack of high-quality studies. Despite years of use with success in patients, the surge in evidence-based medicine has maligned these treatments due to the lack of evidence. However, it should be noted that even some standard therapies lack high-quality evidence, but continue to be used due to tradition. Nonsteroidal anti-inflammatory drug (NSAID) use for chronic tendonitis is one example [1, 2]. But, just because the studies are lacking it does not mean these therapies are not effective. One underlying commonality with all of these complementary treatments is the effect on the fascia through physical intervention. For years, researchers have tried to develop blinded, placebo-controlled, randomized trials. However, trying to develop a placebo for physical intervention like touch or the insertion of an acupuncture needle is difficult. Sham treatments used as placebo still have the physical interaction between patient and practitioner, and may have some effect. Even more difficult is trying to blind the researchers and study subjects to the physical interventions. However, research on the fascia, as well as the biology of manual therapies [3], is giving insight into how it affects muscle function, vascular function, and nerve function. This chapter gives a brief history of complementary medical philosophies and looks at their role in the treatment of posterior lower extremity injury.

Osteopathic Medicine

Andrew Taylor Still, MD, developed osteopathic medicine in the late 1800s in response to seeing and experiencing the limitations and side effects of traditional medicine during his time. He cut ties with the allopathic profession and founded the first school of osteopathic medicine in 1892 in Kirksville, Missouri [4]. Today, the osteopathic philosophy is a "concept of health care supported by expanding scientific knowledge that embraces the concept of the unity of the living organism's structure (anatomy) and function (physiology)" [4]. Osteopathic philosophy emphasizes the following principles: the human being is a dynamic functional unit, the body possesses self-regulatory mechanisms and is self-healing in nature, structure and function are reciprocally

Bo M. Rowan is deceased.

J. B. Dixon (✉)
Sports Medicine, Advanced Center for Orthopedics, Marquette, MI, USA
e-mail: jbryandixon@hotmail.com

interrelated at all levels, and rational treatment is based on these principles [4].

Somatic dysfunction is an impaired or altered function of related components of the somatic system: skeletal, arthrodial, and myofascial structures, and related vascular, lymphatic, and neural elements [5]. This is a very broad term, and can be applied to a wide variety of problems. However, not all somatic lesions are somatic dysfunctions. A somatic dysfunction must be amenable to treatment [5]. Osteopathic manipulative treatments are used to treat somatic dysfunctions that may be impeding the self-regulatory mechanisms. Somatic dysfunction is diagnosed using specific criteria, often abbreviated as TART [5]. This stands for tissue texture change, asymmetry, restriction, and tenderness. Tissue texture changes can be appreciated when soft tissues, including skin, fascia, and muscle, undergo palpable changes. Asymmetry can be appreciated in bones or other structures when one side is compared to the other. Restriction within the bounds of normal physiologic motion, in one or more planes, can be appreciated in the minor motions of a joint. Tenderness on palpation, usually greater than expected for a given area, can be appreciated over areas of somatic dysfunction.

Of course, Still's idea of manual medicine was not new, and his use of spinal manipulation had many precedents [4]. But, it was his organization of these previous concepts into one sound school of thought that made osteopathic medicine stand out among the other alternative medical philosophies of the time. He did not teach his students techniques, but rather urged them to study, test, and improve upon his ideas. Most of the techniques used in osteopathic manipulation were actually developed by his successors. Researchers, notably Irvin Korr, PhD, eventually were able to back up his claims with scientific investigations that provided physiologic evidence of the somatic dysfunction [4]. This eventually distinguished it from its manually based cohorts, chiropractic and naprapathic medicine, which were derived from osteopathic medicine.

Chiropractic Medicine

Chiropractic was founded in 1895 in Davenport, Iowa, by magnetic healer Daniel David Palmer, after studying osteopathy [6]. Chiropractic philosophy includes the perspectives of reductionism, conservatism, and homeostasis [7]. Reductionism in chiropractic reduces causes and cures of health problems to a single factor, vertebral subluxation [8]. Conservatism considers the risks of clinical interventions when balancing them against their benefits. It emphasizes noninvasive treatment to minimize risk, and avoids surgery and medication [9]. Homeostasis emphasizes the body's inherent self-healing abilities. Chiropractic's early notion of innate intelligence can be thought of as a metaphor for homeostasis [10].

Chiropractic theory on spinal joint dysfunction and its putative role in non-musculoskeletal disease has been a source of controversy since its inception in 1895 due to its initial basis in pseudoscience. However, chiropractic medicine has become more respectable since the late twentieth century. Contemporary chiropractors see the value of evidence-based medicine and research into chiropractic treatments. There is evidence that chiropractic spinal manipulation may be useful for low back pain. Some of the manual medicine techniques employed by chiropractors to the posterior lower extremity may also be useful in lower extremity injuries [11].

Naprapathic Medicine

Naprapathic medicine is a specialized system of health care that employs hands-on manual medicine, nutritional counseling, and a wide variety of therapeutic modalities. It was founded in 1908 in Chicago, Illinois, by Oakley Smith, DC, a one-time medical student who had investigated Still's osteopathy in Kirksville, Missouri, before going to study chiropractic under Palmer in Davenport, Iowa.

Naprapathy focuses on conditions caused by impaired myofascial and connective tissue. Connective tissue supports and contains all of the integral structures of the entire body. Conditions may exist where this contracted tissue may impede and create interference with the normal action of nerve pathways, in addition to affecting the proper circulation of blood and lymph. When this occurs, naprapathy contends that the result can be pain, inflammation, and restriction of normal movement of the affected area of the body and negatively affect vessels passing through these tissues [12].

Naprapathic medicine practitioners often use a threefold strategy in the treatment of connective tissue disorders. Naprapathic manual medicine involves gentle connective tissue manipulation to the spine, joints, and articulations of the body. Recommendations are also made for holistic dietary changes and food supplementation, through the use of herbs, vitamins, and minerals, to assist the body in achieving optimal health. Naprapaths also use therapeutic modalities that make use of the effective properties of physical measures of heat, cold, light, water, radiant energy, electricity, sound, air, and assistive devices for the purpose of preventing, correcting, or alleviating a physical disability. Modalities may include ultrasound, electric stimulation, and/or photobiostimulation, also known as low-level laser or cold laser therapy [12].

Traditional Chinese Medicine

TCM is rooted in the ancient philosophy of Taoism and dates back more than 5000 years. The philosophy of TCM is based on the ancient Chinese perception of humans as microcosms of the surrounding universe, interconnected with nature and subject to its forces. The human body is regarded as an organic entity in which the various organs, tissues, and other parts have distinct functions, but are interdependent. In this view, health and disease relate to balance of the functions [13].

The theoretical framework of TCM has a number of key components. Yin-yang theory, which recognizes two opposing, yet complementary forces that shape the world and all life, is central to TCM [13]. TCM also recognizes a vital energy or life force called *qi* (pronounced "chee") that circulates in the body through a system of pathways called meridians. Health is an ongoing process of maintaining balance and harmony in the circulation of qi [13]. The TCM approach uses eight

principles to analyze symptoms and categorize conditions. TCM also uses the theory of five elements to explain how the body works. These elements correspond to particular organs and tissues in the body [13]. TCM practitioners use a variety of therapies in an effort to promote health and treat diseases. The most commonly used are Chinese herbal medicine and acupuncture. Other TCM practices include moxibustion, cupping, massage, mind–body therapy, and dietary therapy [13].

In spite of the widespread use of TCM in China and its use in the West, scientific evidence of its effectiveness is, for the most part, limited. TCM's complexity and underlying conceptual foundations present challenges for researchers seeking evidence on whether and how it works. Most research has focused on specific modalities, primarily acupuncture and Chinese herbal remedies. Acupuncture research has produced a large body of scientific evidence. Studies suggest that it may be useful for a number of different conditions, but additional research is still needed. Chinese herbal medicine has also been studied for a wide range of conditions. Most of the research has been done in China. Although there is evidence that herbs may be effective for some conditions, most studies have been methodologically flawed, and additional, better-designed research is needed before any conclusions can be drawn [13]. Therefore, this chapter will only discuss acupuncture techniques.

Common Themes

All of the above medical philosophies share some commonalities, likely due to the fact that with the exception of TCM, they were all developed in close geographical and temporal proximity to one another. All of them view the body as a unit with interconnected parts that are interrelated while functioning independently, ascertain that lesions in one part of the body can affect flow of substances to other parts of the body, and that manipulation of the body can resolve the lesions, normalize the flow of substances, and restore the body's normal function to improve health. Another commonality is that despite the lack of published studies indicating effectiveness, practitioners in each of these professions have treated patients with success for the past hundred-plus years in the case of osteopathic, chiropractic, and naprapathic; and for thousands of years in the case of TCM. Even more telling, patients continue to turn to these complementary treatments when traditional Western medicine, often termed *allopathic,* cannot treat pain effectively.

The difference between each of the philosophies rests in the focus of the manipulations and the substance being targeted. TCM focuses on manipulating qi and improving the flow of this energy through the body. Osteopathic medicine focuses on manipulating bones, joints, muscles, nerves, and fascia to improve vascular flow, including lymphatics. Chiropractic medicine focused on manipulating the spine to improve nerve function. Naprapathic medicine focuses on manipulating ligaments, tendons, and the related muscles and fascia to restore the body's normal movement. Despite the superficial difference in the focal point of treatment modalities, there is one underlying theme—fascia.

Fascia

Fascia is the connective tissue that unites all aspects of the body, and although previously thought to just function as packing tissue or a cushion to organs, fascia is now being thought of as a separate organ system involved in tissue protection and the healing of surrounding systems [14, 15]. All of the philosophies mentioned above affect the fascia in some way, as fascia covers everything including nerves, blood vessels, lymphatic vessels, bones, muscles, tendons, and ligaments. It is like the technique is the dart, and the fascia is the board. Many of the techniques used in each profession are very similar, and there is a lot of crossover of techniques between all practitioners of manual medicine.

Neuropathic Pain

Neuropathic pain results from a disturbance in neurologic function, which may or may not correspond to any apparent pathology in the peripheral nerves [16]. Signs of neuropathy include sensory, motor, or autonomic dysfunction in the dermatome, myotome, or sclerotome [17]. Clinical presentation may include absence of obvious damaged tissue, delayed onset of signs and symptoms, abnormal sensations, a deep, aching pain or shooting, stabbing pain, pain in a region of sensory deficit, allodynia, diminished range of motion, and/or pain upon muscle contraction [16]. Neuropathic pain may be amenable to intramuscular stimulation through dry needling techniques [16, 18].

Myofascial Pain

Investigations to find the cause of persistent pain in the posterior lower leg are usually directed at excluding diseases of the bones or joints, circulatory disorders, and neuropathies. The possibility that myofascial disruption is the cause of the pain is often missed initially [19]. Travell and Simons initially described trigger points as the cause of myofascial pain [15, 16, 20–22]. These consist of hyperirritable points in the muscle or fascial layers that are neurologically maintained through facilitation, and often involve autonomic nervous system findings. They can be influenced by stress from physiological as well as psychological origins [16, 20].

A muscle with a trigger point has a diminished range of motion and diminished strength due to pain and neurologic factors [16]. Trigger points are identified as a localized spot of tenderness within a muscle knot, associated with a palpable taut band of muscle fibers, or possibly a slight tremor [20]. Applying pressure to the trigger point reproduces the patient's pain pattern or a part of their pain pattern [20]. A local twitch response may be elicited when a snapping, shearing stress, like plucking a guitar string, is applied across the taut band [16]. Active trigger points are noticeably painful even without palpation. Latent trigger points typically are only painful on palpation, but may become activated. Postural imbalances, overuse, local injury or other stimuli like the cooling of tired, immobile legs by an air-conditioned automobile, for example, may cause a latent trigger point to become activated [16, 21].

The etiology of trigger points is best explained by the integrated energy crisis and motor end-plate hypotheses [21, 23, 24]. In addition, noxious substances in muscles with active trigger points have been found which stimulate nocireceptors as well as cause an acidic environment [25, 26], adding strength to the integrated hypothesis [23]. The most common cause of trigger points may be poor posture causing sustained stress in muscles [27]. Trigger points may also be caused by muscle overload, as a result of trauma or overuse/repetitive stress injuries, and immobilization may sustain them [16]. Lower extremity ischemia may also activate trigger points. Extrinsic causes of decreased blood flow to the lower extremity might include sustained compression from long socks with a tight elastic band at the top, a cast that is too tight, or a chair with a high front edge. All of these can compress the soft tissues and decrease blood flow to the lower extremity [16]. Additionally, one study showed that a factor contributing to the pain of intermittent claudication is the activation of trigger points in the gastrocnemius and soleus, when these muscles become ischemic as a result of decreased blood supply to the leg [19]. They further showed that deactivating these trigger points, by injecting procaine into them, increases the exercise capacity of the limb in spite of the limited blood flow to the limb. Deactivation of the trigger points in these two muscles is therefore a worthwhile therapeutic procedure in this condition, and one that can be done more readily and just as effectively by inserting dry needles into the tissues overlying the trigger points [19]. Acute trigger points become chronic trigger points if not treated. Chronic trigger points are complicated by further neurological involvement, become more painful, and are more difficult to treat [16]. Therefore, considering causes of trigger points as part of the initial evaluation of posterior lower extremity pain, and looking for trigger points, is essential.

Posterior Lower Extremity Trigger Points

Activities that require forceful plantar flexion at the ankle with the knee bent, such as climbing steep slopes, jogging uphill, or riding a bike with the seat too low, may activate trigger points by overloading the gastrocnemius and/or soleus [16]. Other activities might be walking on hard, slick surfaces with flat shoes that cause slippage of the forefoot during the push-off phase of the gait, or prolonged activity to which the patient is unaccustomed. Walking on a graded slope or domed street or standing while leaning for a prolonged period are other examples of activities that may cause trigger points [16]. Wearing a heel that is too high or a unilateral heel lift that is too large may be a cause of chronic overuse. Other characteristics of posterior lower extremity trigger points are listed in Table 13.1.

Gastrocnemius trigger points become activated in the belly of the muscle in the center of the calf as a result of the muscle becoming strained, either as a primary event, or when a limp develops as a result of a painful disorder occurring in the heel or foot, and also when, because of a circulatory disorder, the muscle becomes ischemic. Pain from the trigger points in this muscle is felt in the calf and the sole of the foot. It is often worse when walking uphill, and may be associated with the development of nocturnal cramps, often misdiagnosed as restless leg syndrome [19]. Figure 13.1 shows the locations of the gastrocnemius trigger points.

The soleus is liable to develop trigger points in its distal third for the same reasons as they develop in the gastrocnemius. Pain from these trigger points is referred distally along the Achilles tendon to the heel. The pain may also be referred upwards to the ipsilateral sacroiliac joint. The posterior part of the gluteus minimus can also refer pain to the calf, and this can activate satellite trigger points to the soleus [16]. The ankle jerk reflex may be decreased or absent in patients with trigger points in the soleus. The deactivation of the trigger points restores this reflex to normal [19]. A small study showed a significant improvement in ankle range of motion after a single intervention on latent soleus trigger points [28]. It is particularly important to distinguish between pain developing in the base of the heel as a result of an inflammatory lesion in the tendon, and pain referred to that site from trigger points in the soleus muscle. In Achilles tendonitis, the

Table 13.1 Characteristics of trigger points in the posterior lower extremity

Muscle	Activation/perpetuation	Symptoms	Examination
Gastrocnemius	Muscle overload/prolonged plantar flexion	Nocturnal calf cramps	Restriction of knee extension with ankle in dorsiflexion
Soleus	Muscle overload, forefoot slipping/prolonged plantar flexion	Heel pain and tenderness	Restriction of ankle dorsiflexion with knee in flexion, Achilles reflex may be reduced
Plantaris	Muscle overload, forefoot slipping/prolonged plantar flexion	Posterior knee and upper calf pain	Restriction of ankle dorsiflexion with knee in flexion, Achilles reflex may be reduced
Popliteus	Running, twisting, or sliding with knee bent	Posterior knee pain with knee bent	Passive lateral rotation restricted by pain with thigh fixed and knee flexed at 90°
Tibialis posterior	Chronic muscle overload, jogging on uneven surfaces/prolonged hyperpronation	Pain in sole, arch, or Achilles tendon while walking or running	Functional weakness, restricted ROM, aching pain when muscle is actively retracted in fully shortened position
Long toe flexors (FHL, FDL)	Running on uneven ground/walking, running on soft sand, Morton foot structure, prolonged hyperpronation	Painful feet, especially with weight bearing	Weakness in toe flexion, restricted ROM in extension

ROM range of motion, *FHL* flexor hallucis longus, *FDL* flexor digitorum longus

Fig. 13.1 Gastrocnemius trigger points *(X)* and pain referral patterns *(red color)*. *Solid color* is primary site of pain, with *stippling* indicating the spillover pattern. **a** Trigger point 1, **b** trigger point 2, **c** trigger point 3, **d** trigger point 4

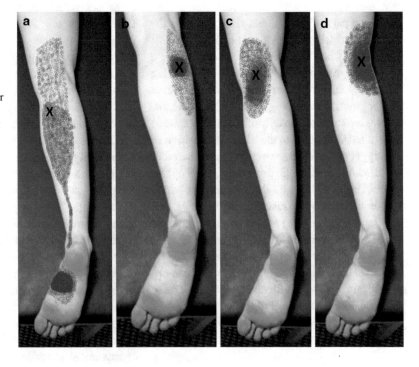

tendon is liable to be slightly swollen and there may be crepitus over it when the foot is moved. On examination, exquisitely tender trigger points are found in the tissues around the tendon. Inserting dry needles in the tissues overlying these trigger points may relieve the pain. This usually has to be repeated three or more times at weekly intervals in order to obtain any lasting benefit,

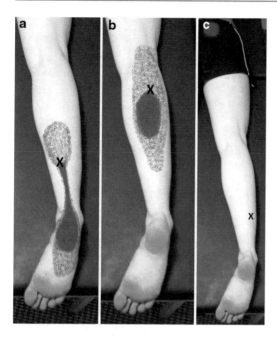

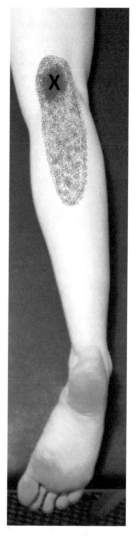

Fig. 13.3 Plantaris trigger point *(X)* and pain referral pattern *(red color)*. *Solid color* is primary site of pain, with *stippling* indicating the spillover pattern

Fig. 13.2 Soleus trigger points *(X)* and pain referral patterns *(red color)*. *Solid color* is primary site of pain, with *stippling* indicating the spillover pattern. **a** Trigger point 1, **b** trigger point 2, **c** trigger point 3

but is certainly preferable to steroid injection at this site. The steroid injection is associated with much postinjection pain, and if inadvertently injected into the tendon sheath, may cause rupture of the tendon, requiring surgical repair [19]. Figure 13.2 shows the locations of the soleus trigger points.

Plantaris trigger points are commonly associated with soleus tender points [27]. They primarily refer pain to the back of the knee as well, with pain extending about midway down the back of the calf [27]. Figure 13.3 shows the location of the plantaris trigger point.

Popliteus trigger points primarily refer pain to the back of the knee joint. Pain may be worse with crouching, going downhill or downstairs. There is rarely pain at night [27]. These trigger points may be associated with gastrocnemius and plantaris trigger points [27]. Figure 13.4 shows the location of the popliteus trigger point.

Tibialis posterior trigger points concentrate proximally over the Achilles tendon above the heel, but may extend from the trigger point down over the calf, the entire heel, and the plantar surface of the foot and toes [27]. The trigger points in the tibialis posterior may be indirectly palpated through other muscles. Interpreting tenderness at this site depends on the preceding examination establishing involvement of this muscle and determining that the surrounding muscles are free of tenderness [27]. Figure 13.5 shows the location of the tibialis posterior trigger point.

The long toe flexors, flexor hallucis longus (FHL) and flexor digitorum longus (FDL) help to control motions of the foot. Trigger points may become activated in situations where the foot is unstable [27]. Pain referred from the FDL is felt in the middle of the plantar forefoot proximal to

Fig. 13.4 cating the spillover patternPopliteus trigger point *(X)* and pain referral pattern *(red color)*. *Solid color* is primary site of pain, with *stippling* indi

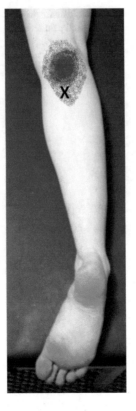

Fig. 13.5 Tibialis posterior trigger point *(X)* and pain referral pattern *(red color)*. *Solid color* is primary site of pain, with *stippling* indicating the spillover pattern

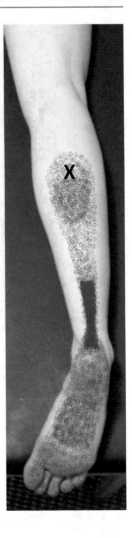

the lateral digits. Pain referred from the FHL is felt in the plantar surface of the great toe and head of the first metatarsal [27]. Figure 13.6 shows the locations of the long toe flexor trigger points.

Trigger Point Treatment

Treatment is typically done with injection of a local anesthetic or dry needling, either with a small-gauge hypodermic needle or an acupuncture needle. Injections using preservative-free products are generally recommended to minimize the damage produced by the anesthetic [16]. This is consistent with the goal of minimizing neurological irritation.

The patient positions for gastrocnemius trigger injections are lateral recumbent on the ipsilateral side for trigger point 1, on the contralateral side for trigger point 2, and prone for trigger points 3 and 4. Using a pincer grasp on the trigger points, insert a 27-gauge 1.5-in. needle directly into trigger point 1 and trigger point 2 without

worry of neurovascular structures. Injection of trigger point 3 and trigger point 4 must proceed with caution, and the needle should be directed away from the midline. The trigger points can be infiltrated with 0.5 mL of Marcaine 0.25%, and this can be done with a multi-quadrant approach for trigger point 1 and trigger point 2 [16].

The patient positions for soleus trigger point injections are lateral recumbent on the ipsilateral side for trigger points 1 and 2, and on the contralateral side for trigger point 3. Using a pincer grasp on trigger point 1 and trigger point 3, insert a 27-gauge 1.5-in. needle into trigger point 1 through a medial approach and into trigger point 3 through a lateral approach. For injection of trigger point 2, the needle is directed toward the fibula, because the trigger point is close to the

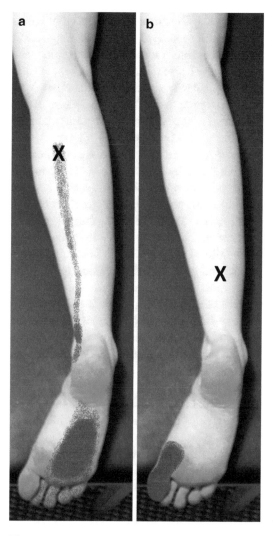

Fig. 13.6 Long toe flexor trigger points *(X)* and pain referral patterns *(red color)*. *Solid color* is primary site of pain, with *stippling* indicating the spillover pattern. The flexor digitorum longus point (**a**) is pictured on the *left*, the flexor hallucis longus point (**b**) is pictured on the *right*

bone. The trigger points can be infiltrated with 0.5 mL of Marcaine 0.25 %. This can be done in a multi-quadrant approach for trigger point 1 and trigger point 2 [16].

Trigger point injection may result in soreness for 5–6 days afterward. The stretching exercises help to relieve this, but as a precaution you may only want to treat one side in a visit. The patient may also use acetaminophen for residual pain after the injection [16, 27]. Muscle retraining

exercise and maintenance exercises are recommended after treatment [16].

Acupuncture/Dry Needling

The precise origin of acupuncture is a source of debate. Evidence exists for a variety of potential antecedent practices [29]. Even today, there is no standardized approach to acupuncture due to past acupuncture scholars freely editing prior texts [29]. Classic acupuncture refers to thin, solid metallic needles inserted into the skin at specific points along meridians that correspond to internal organs. This is done to restore the balance in the body. In traditional Chinese acupuncture, needle effectiveness is frequently measured by the elicitation of de qi. The patient may feel a throbbing ache, while the practitioner feels a grasp of the needle by the tissue [29]. One proposed theory is that acupuncture points are associated with anatomic locations of loose connective tissue. Studies have shown a relationship between fascial structures and acupuncture points and meridians, as well as a relationship between connective tissue and the effects of acupuncture [30–33]. One study has also shown a decrease in alpha-motoneuron activity after acupuncture [34]. When combined with the theories behind myofascial pain, acupuncture may have a role in treating pain associated with posterior lower extremity injuries.

Trigger points may be treated with acupuncture techniques including dry needling and intramuscular stimulation. A number 3 (0.2 mm by 40 mm) acupuncture needle is used. The patient position for treatments is prone. The trigger point(s) are identified. The acupuncture needle is placed perpendicular to the skin into the trigger point. The practitioner depresses the skin firmly with the insertion tube to cause a local anesthetic effect, then taps the needle through the skin barrier. The tube is removed and the needle directed toward the trigger point in a pecking/probing manner. The practitioner should proceed with caution for blood vessels and nerves that lie in the midline. Ideally, there will be muscle twitching in response to this procedure, as well as a grab of the needle by the muscle. This grab is usually released instantaneously [16]. The needle may be rotated until the patient feels a dull throbbing at the point. The procedure is terminated when the discomfort level is 7/10 per patient, or if there is no muscle grab and the muscle seems to have relaxed [16]. In some cases, there is a strong spasm of the muscle during treatment. In this case, the needle can be left in place for 10–20 min, without manipulating the needle, before removal. The spasm is not usually accompanied by pain unless the needle is manipulated during the spasm [16].

Muscle Energy

Muscle energy is a technique that may be used following trigger point treatments [16]. It was developed by Fred L. Mitchell, Sr., DO, although similar techniques were previously described [35]. There are nine different physiologic principles that may be used in muscle energy [35], although post-isometric relaxation may be the most common one used. The physiologic basis behind this principle is that immediately after isometric contraction, the neuromuscular apparatus is in a refractory state allowing for passive stretching to be performed without encountering strong myotactic reflex opposition [35]. Generally, the practitioner positions the patient's body so that the muscle is at its pathological barrier. The patient pushes about 5 pounds of force against that barrier for 5 s while contracting the muscle (isometric contraction). Upon relaxing, the physician follows the relaxation to engage a new barrier reflecting the lengthened muscle. This is repeated 3–5 times or until the range of motion stops improving. If there is no release toward a new barrier, then the dysfunction is likely not of muscular origin, and the diagnosis should be reconsidered [16]. The post-contraction relaxation period prevents stretch receptors from activating [3], allowing for increased stretch in the muscle and increased range of motion at restricted joints.

The muscles of the posterior lower extremity can be treated with the patient prone and knee extended with their feet hanging off the end of the table. Dorsiflexion at the patient's foot is controlled and encouraged through the physician's leg or knee contact on the forefoot, to the point of the initial barrier. The patient is instructed to apply a plantar flexion force against the physician's resistance for 5 s. Upon relaxation after the 5-s force the foot is dorsiflexed further into the new barrier. This is repeated 3–5 times or until no further barrier is appreciated. Ice or vapocoolant spray may be applied in a proximal to distal direction along the calf. This should be done after the initial plantar flexion to the barrier [16]. Treatment can also be done with the patient prone and knee flexed. Dorsiflexion at the patient's foot is controlled and encouraged through the physician's hand contact on the forefoot, to the point of the initial barrier. The patient is instructed to apply a plantar flexion force against the physician's resistance for 5 s. Upon relaxation after the 5-s force the foot is dorsiflexed further into the new barrier. This is repeated 3–5 times or until no further barrier is appreciated. Cool and stretch may be used in this position also.

After cool and stretch, the muscle may be rewarmed with a heating pack for 5–10 min. After rewarming, the patient is instructed to move through their greatest range of motion [16]. Ideally, the patient should not return to previous activities immediately afterward, as the muscle needs a period of rest. Patients can attain the most benefit if they soak the muscle in a hot bath as soon as possible and practice the prescribed stretches. As the muscle fibers are allowed to relax, they release toxins, which may result in discomfort that the patient identifies as similar to the pretreatment pain. Stretching wrings the toxins out of the muscle and may result in immediate alleviation of posttreatment discomfort [16].

Strain–Counterstrain

This technique was developed by Lawrence H. Jones, DO, as a treatment for tender points in the muscle belly. These tender points can occur due to chemical or mechanical sensitization causing an increase in afferent flow [36–38]. Edema and increased muscular pressure may also induce

Table 13.2 Comparison of tender points and trigger points

Tender point	Trigger point
No characteristic pain pattern	Characteristic pain pattern
Located in muscle, tendons, ligaments, and fascia	Located in muscle tissue
Locally tender	Locally tender
Elicits jump sign when pressed	Elicits jump sign when pressed
No radiating pattern when pressed	Elicits a radiating pain pattern when pressed
Taut band not present	Present within a taut band of tissue
Twitch response not present	Elicits twitch response with snapping palpation
Dermographia not present	Dermographia of skin over point

these points locally in the muscle belly, but these points may be perpetuated by long-term changes in the synaptic processes in dorsal horn neurons [36]. These tender points share some characteristics with trigger points, but can be differentiated clinically (Table 13.2) and are still separated in the literature [38].

Treatment consists of first identifying a tender point. This helps to determine which muscle is dysfunctional, as well as the position of treatment. Once identified, a pain scale is established with the patient, with the pain felt on palpation of the tender point being a 10/10. The physician then approximates the origin and the insertion of the dysfunctional muscle until the patient's pain is reduced by 70 % (3/10 or less). This position is held for at least 90 s, during which the physician monitors the point but does not need to apply pressure. This allows the muscle spindle, alpha, and gamma nerves to return to their normal balance from a hyperactive state [3, 16, 36–38]. Then the patient is slowly, passively returned to the neutral position. The physician rechecks the tender point to ensure successful treatment after the patient is returned to neutral. The slow return to neutral is essential, as the dysfunctional muscle is still neurochemically sensitive and must be given a day or two of rest to achieve a new neurologic balance. Patients should be instructed to hold off on prescribed stretches or any intense activity for 1–2 days after counterstrain treatment. This treatment is tolerated well by patients, requires no additional equipment, and is effective for both acute and chronic pain [38]. If pain remains, the treatment may be repeated. If the treatment is not successful after several attempts, the diagnosis should be reconsidered.

Myofascial Release

Myofascial release is a system of diagnosis and treatment originating with A. T. Still and his students, which engages continual palpatory feedback to achieve release of myofascial tissue [39]. The techniques are a group of specific maneuvers that generally achieve the same goal of myofascial release. They can be used as the primary treatment modality, in combination with each other, or in combination with other modalities [40]. The techniques and mechanism of action are described elsewhere [39]. Direct methods may be used, in which the fascia is taken into the restriction until a release is felt; or indirect methods may be used, in which the fascia is taken into the position of comfort until a release is felt. Acute injuries may be better treated using the indirect methods for patient comfort. Chronic injuries may be treated with direct or indirect methods depending on patient's comfort.

The effects of the techniques on homeostasis include relaxation of contracted muscles, increased circulation to an ischemic area, increased venous and lymphatic drainage, and a stimulatory effect of the stretch reflex on hypotonic muscles [40]. This ultimately decreases the oxygen demand of the muscle, increases oxygen supply to the muscle, increases the removal of harmful metabolic waste products, and mobilizes fluid. This can help the healing process in musculoskeletal injuries by breaking the pain-tension-pain cycle and preventing a fibrous reaction, which causes fascial shortening and limits muscle stretch and joint mobility [40].

Although no studies looking specifically at myofascial release techniques were found for the lower leg, this modality definitely has a place in the treatment of posterior lower extremity injuries. It is a popular modality among athletic trainers and sports medicine providers, osteopathic physicians, and other manual medicine providers. It is useful for both acute and chronic injuries.

Massage/Soft Tissue Techniques

The benefits of massage on soft tissues are well known. Massage is commonly used to release myofascial tension and improve vascular flow. However, there may be differences between a general massage and a massage given with a specific goal. In one study, there was a modest improvement in ankle dorsiflexion using specific myofascial receptor massage techniques in the distal myotendinous junction of the calf compared to using classical massage techniques on the belly of the calf muscles [41]. This difference was seen immediately after treatment, but seemed to have an even greater effect 10 min after treatment.

Ligamentous Articular Strain

William G. Sutherland, DO, primarily devised this technique. It is also known as the balanced ligamentous tension technique. It is based on the idea that ligamentous tension in joints has little variation due to the fact that ligaments do not stretch and contract like muscles [42]. In normal movements, the relationship between a joint's ligaments changes as the joint changes position, but the total tension in the ligamentous articular mechanism does not. However, when injury, inflammation, or mechanical stressors affect the joint, the distribution of the tension between the ligaments is altered [42]. This altered tension can have an effect elsewhere in the kinetic chain, as the fascia that comprises the affected ligaments arises from the muscles on either side of the affected joint. The goal of this modality is to restore the normal balance in the ligamentous tension in order to restore normal function—locally through joint physiology, and remotely through the fascia and fluid dynamics [42].

The principles of this technique are disengagement, exaggeration, and balance. The practitioner first compresses or decompresses the joint or fascial plane, and increases the pressure or traction until the practitioner is able to passively move the injured part. Then the injured part is passively moved back to the original injury position until a point of balance is found. This balanced position is maintained until a release in the tissue is appreciated, and structures return to their normal functional positions [42].

Although not as common, and therefore not as well studied as some of the other osteopathic modalities, this technique is relatively safe and the risks to the patient are minimal when done correctly. It may have a place for pain refractory to other treatment modalities. Further studies evaluating its effectiveness in injuries to the posterior lower extremity are needed.

Prolotherapy

Prolotherapy is a technique in which a proliferent solution is injected into a ligament in order to stimulate collagen production and strengthen the ligament, particularly at sites of bony attachment. It has been in use as a treatment for chronic musculoskeletal pain since the 1930s [43]. Despite its increasing popularity as a treatment for ligament and joint laxity, conclusive data is lacking [43]. However, the effectiveness of prolotherapy seems to be operator-dependent, and this may not be reflected in the selection of study subjects, skewing the results away from a positive effect if there is one [43]. In the hands of an experienced operator, prolotherapy may be a possible treatment option for certain patients, but studies in the lower extremity have been limited to looking at the effects of this treatment on the knee [43].

Transdermal Techniques

The transdermal techniques used in musculoskeletal injuries include cryotherapy, electrical stimulation, laser therapy, ultrasound, iontophoresis, magnets, and topical preparations. These methods are commonly used to treat acute pain after injury or prevent secondary muscle injury due to inflammation, edema, and/or ischemia.

Cryotherapy, using ice or chemical cold packs or cold water baths, can decrease regional blood flow and hemorrhage, decrease edema, reduce inflammation, and induce analgesia [44, 45]. Studies have shown that cryotherapy may reduce postexercise muscle damage, but did not find an effect on perception of pain or weakness [44, 46]. This is a safe and inexpensive method for treatment of muscle injuries.

Electrical stimulation, most commonly with transcutaneous electrical nerve stimulation (TENS) units, is considered safe with a low risk of complications. There is evidence that use of electrical stimulation produces pain scores in traumatic and overuse injuries, pain due to peripheral nerve damage, and pain due to mechanical causes [47, 48], but further studies looking at the effect of electrical stimulation on muscle function are needed [44].

Low-level laser therapy is tolerated well, with few risks or contraindications. It is commonly used for acute and overuse injuries; however, it is expensive compared to other modalities. Its effectiveness for analgesia in musculoskeletal conditions needs further study [44, 49, 50].

Ultrasound therapies, including phonophoresis and extracorporeal shockwave therapy (ESWT), are another popular modality used for soft tissue injuries. Ultrasound by itself produces a thermal effect on the tissues that increases blood flow and soft tissue extensibility. It also has nonthermal effects, namely cavitation, which can promote wound healing, but has a less clear role in musculoskeletal injuries [44, 51, 52]. The studies on the use of ultrasound for musculoskeletal injuries are mixed for use in delayed-onset muscle soreness [44, 53–55]. Studies show little evidence for use in soft tissue injury [56] or for analgesia in musculoskeletal injuries [57]. ESWT uses high energy focused ultrasound energy to induce tissue changes. It may be useful in calcific tendinopathy in certain joints, but there is no evidence it is useful in chronic or noncalcific tendinopathies, or in the lower extremity [1]. Further studies are needed.

Phonophoresis, a process by which pharmacologic agents are driven transdermally into subcutaneous tissues with ultrasound, has little support in the literature [44, 55, 58]. Iontophoresis, which is similar to phonophoresis except that electrical current is used instead of ultrasound, does have support in the literature for reducing acute pain in certain areas [44, 59, 60], but further studies on its effectiveness in the posterior lower leg need to be done.

Magnets are inexpensive, safe, and popular among athletes and nonathletes for their presumed healing power. There is evidence that magnet therapy can reduce inflammation [61], as well as influence nerve function [44, 62]. However, magnets have not been shown to reduce pain in properly designed studies [44, 62, 63]. Continued studies are recommended.

Topical preparations, like capsaicin or NSAIDs, are easily used and generally well tolerated. However, local reactions can occur at the site of application, and topical NSAIDs can rarely cause systemic effects [44, 64, 65]. There is good evidence that capsaicin is useful for osteoarthritic knee pain [66], but its use in acute sports injuries has not been described [44]. Topical NSAIDs have shown some benefit for relief of pain, but there is little evidence for improvement in muscle function after injury [44, 67]. Dimethyl sulfoxide (DMSO) has not shown benefit in studies [44].

Hyperbaric Oxygen

Hyperbaric oxygen (HBO) therapy is recommended as adjunctive therapy for a range of traumatic and ischemic syndromes [68, 69]. HBO is thought to work through several mechanisms including increasing tissue oxygenation, reducing edema through hyperoxia-induced vasospasm, reducing the inflammatory response, enhancing collagen deposition, inhibiting the release of oxygen free radicals, and protecting from reperfusion injury and secondary ischemia [69–72]. Anecdotal evidence suggests that soft tissue injuries may benefit from HBO, but well-designed studies have failed to show any beneficial effect for ankle sprains or delayed-onset muscle soreness [73–75]. Further well-designed studies are recommended.

Summary

Complementary therapies have been around for many years. The science behind the treatments is finally starting to catch up. Researchers are discovering reasons for why these therapies may work, especially with regard to manual therapies that target the fascia. Continued research is needed, as many of these treatments are still working on basic science theory, and have not yet shown any clinically significant difference. Despite this, these complementary treatments should not be dismissed immediately, as patients may find relief with one or more of the modalities. As with all medicine, having the patient make an informed decision should be the goal for practitioners. Presenting the patient with the option of complementary therapies, and explaining the risks, benefits, and limitations including possible failure of the therapy will help them make an informed decision.

References

1. Andres BM, Murrell GA. Treatment of tendinopathy: what works, what does not, and what is on the horizon. Clin Orthop Relat Res. 2008;466(7):1539–54.
2. Rees JD, Wilson AM, Wolman RL. Current concepts in the management of tendon disorders. Rheumatology (Oxford). 2006;45(5):508–21.
3. Clark BC, Thomas JS, Walkowski SA, Howell JN. The biology of manual therapies. J Am Osteopath Assoc. 2012;112(9):617–29.
4. Seffinger MA, King HH, Ward RC, Jones JM, Rogers FJ, Patterson MM. Osteopathic philosophy. In: Chila AG, editor. Foundations of osteopathic medicine. 3rd ed. Philadelphia: Lippincott Williams & Wilkins; 2011. p. 3–22.
5. DiGiovanna EL. Somatic dysfunction. In: DiGiovanna EL, Schiowits S, editors. An osteopathic approach to diagnosis and treatment. 2nd ed. Philadelphia: Lippincott Williams & Wilkins; 1997. p. 7–12.
6. Leach R. The chiropractic theories: a textbook of scientific research. Philadelphia: Lippincott Williams & Wilkins; 2004.
7. Mootz RD, Phillips RB. Chiropractic belief systems. In: Cherkin DC, Mootz RD, editors. Chiropractic in the United States: training, practice, and research. Rockville: Agency for Health Care Policy and Research; 1997. p. 9–16.
8. Murphy DR, Schneider MJ, Seaman DR, Perle SM, Nelson CF. How can chiropractic become a respected mainstream profession? The example of podiatry. Chiropr Osteopat. 2008;16:10.
9. American Chiropractic Association [homepage on the Internet]. History of chiropractic care. Arlington, VA; The Association; 2013. (cited 2013 Jun 1). http://www.acatoday.org/level3_css.cfm?T1ID=13&T2ID=61&T3ID=149.
10. Keating JC Jr. Philosophy in chiropractic. In: Haldeman S, Dagenais S, Budgell B et al., editors. Principles and practice of chiropractic. 3rd ed. New York: McGraw-Hill; 2005. p. 77–98.
11. Rinn TB, Nelson RC. Medial gastrocnemius tear ("tennis leg"): a case report. Chiropr Sports Med. 1996;10(1):37–40.
12. American Naprapathic Association [homepage on the Internet]. Oswego, IL. The association; 2013. (cited 2013 Jun 1). http://www.naprapathy.org.
13. Berman B, Ge A, Khalsa P, editors. Traditional Chinese medicine: An introduction. National center for complementary and alternative medicine, national institutes of health, U.S department of health and human services. 2009. (updated 2010, cited 2013 Jun 1):1–8. http://nccam.nih.gov/health/whatiscam/chinesemed.htm.
14. Willard FH, Fossum C, Standley PR. The fascial system of the body. In: Chila AG, editor. Foundations of osteopathic medicine. 3rd ed. Philadelphia: Lippincott Williams & Wilkins; 2011. p. 74–92.
15. O'Connell JA. Bioelectric fascial activation and release: the physician's guide to hunting with Dr. Still. Indianapolis: American Academy of Osteopathy; 1998.
16. Danto JB. Normalization of muscle function: a holistic approach to the diagnosis & treatment of muscle pain & dysfunction. West Bloomfield: Samjill Publishing Company, LLC; 2005.
17. Bonica JJ. The management of pain. 2nd ed. Media: Williams & Wilkins; 1990.
18. Gunn CC. The Gunn approach to the treatment of chronic pain: intramuscular stimulation for myofascial pain of radiculopathic origin. New York: Churchill Livingston; 1999.
19. Baldry PE. Acupuncture, trigger points and musculoskeletal pain. 3rd ed. Philadelphia: Elsevier; 2005.
20. DiGiovanna JA. Trigger point therapy. In: DiGiovanna EL, Schiowits S, editors. An osteopathic approach to diagnosis and treatment. 2nd ed. Philadelphia: Lippincott Williams & Wilkins; 1997. p. 479–81.
21. Huguenin LK. Myofascial trigger points: the current evidence. Phys Ther Sport. 2004;5:2–12.
22. Huguenin LK. Therapies for myofascial trigger points. In: Tiidus PM, editor. Skeletal muscle damage and repair. Champaign: Human Kinetics; 2008. p. 245–55.
23. Simons DG. New views of myofascial trigger points: etiology and diagnosis. Arch Phys Med Rehabil. 2008;89:157–9.
24. Simons DG. Review of enigmatic MTrPs as a common cause of enigmatic musculoskeletal pain and dysfunction. J Electromyogr Kinesiol. 2004;14:95–107.
25. Shah JP, Phillips TM, Danoff JV, Gerber LH. An in vivo micro-analytical technique for measuring the local biochemical milieu of human skeletal muscle. J Appl Physiol. 2005;99:1977–84.

26. Shah JP, Danoff JV, Desai MJ, Parikh S, Nakamura LY, Phillips TM, et al. Biochemicals associated with pain and inflammation are elevated in sites near to and remote from active myofascial trigger points. Arch Phys Med Rehabil. 2008;89:16–23.

27. Travell JG, Simons DG. Myofascial pain and dysfunction: the trigger point manual. Vol. 2. Philadelphia: Lippincott Williams & Wilkins; 1993.

28. Grieve R, Clark J, Pearson E, Bullock S, Boyer C, Jarrett A. The immediate effect of soleus trigger point pressure release on restricted ankle dorsiflexion: a pilot randomised controlled trial. J Bodyw Mov Ther. 2011;15:42–9.

29. Ahn AC. Acupuncture. In: UpToDate, Post TW (Ed), UpToDate, Waltham, MA. Accessed on April 1, 2013.

30. Langevin HM, Yandow JA. Relationship of acupuncture points and meridians to connective tissue planes. Anat Rec. 2002;269:257.

31. Langevin HM, Churchill DL, Wu J, Badger GJ, Yandow JA, Fox JR, et al. Evidence of connective tissue involvement in acupuncture. FASEB J. 2002;16:872.

32. Langevin HM, Churchill DL, Cipolla MJ. Mechanical signaling through connective tissue: a mechanism for the therapeutic effect of acupuncture. FASEB J. 2001;15:2275.

33. Moncayo R, Rudisch A, Kremser C, Moncayo H. 3D-MRI rendering of the anatomical structures related to acupuncture points of the Dai mai, Yin qiao mai and Yang qiao mai meridians within the context of the WOMED concept of lateral tension: implications for musculoskeletal disease. BMC Musculoskelet Disord. 2007;8:33. doi:10.1186/1471-2474-8-33. (Published online 2007 April 10).

34. Chan AK, Vujnovich A, Bradnam-Roberts L. The effect of acupuncture on alpha-motoneuron excitability. Acupunct Electrother Res. 2004;29(1–2):53–72.

35. Ehrenfeuchter WC. Muscle energy approach. In: Chila AG, editor. Foundations of osteopathic medicine. 3rd ed. Philadelphia: Lippincott Williams & Wilkins; 1997. p. 683–97.

36. Rennie PR. Counterstrain and exercise: an integrated approach. 3rd ed. Henderson: RennieMatrix; 2012.

37. Jones LH. Jones strain-counterstrain. Boise: Jones Strain-Counterstrain, Inc.; 1995.

38. Glover JC, Rennie PR. Strain and counterstrain approach. In: Chila AG, editor. Foundations of osteopathic medicine. 3rd ed. Philadelphia: Lippincott Williams & Wilkins; 1997. p. 749–62.

39. O'Connell JA. Myofascial release approach. In: Chila AG, editor. Foundations of osteopathic medicine. 3rd ed. Philadelphia: Lippincott Williams & Wilkins; 1997. p. 698–727.

40. Spinaris T, DiGiovanna EL. Myofascial techniques. In: DiGiovanna EL, Schiowitz S, editors. An osteopathic approach to diagnosis and treatment. 2nd ed. Philadelphia: Lippincott Wiliams & Wilkins; 1997. p. 83–5.

41. Berglund O, Brunberg M, Skillgate E, Viklund P. Comparison of ankle joint dorsiflexion after classical massage or specific myofascial receptor massage technique on the calf muscle [abstract]. Vancouver: Third International Fascia Research Congress; 2012.

42. Crow WT. Balanced ligamentous tension and ligamentous articular strain. In: Chila AG, editor. Foundations of osteopathic medicine. 3rd ed. Philadelphia: Lippincott Williams & Wilkins; 1997. p. 809–13.

43. Rabago D, Best TM, Beamsley M, Patterson J. A systematic review of prolotherapy for chronic musculoskeletal pain. Clin J Sport Med. 2005;15(5):376–80.

44. Bolin DJ. Transdermal approaches to pain in sports injury management. Curr Sports Med Rep. 2003;2:303–9.

45. Knight KL. Cryotherapy: theory, technique, and physiology. Chattanooga: Chattanooga Corporation; 1985.

46. Eston R, Peters D. Effects of cold water immersion on the symptoms of exercise-induced muscle damage. J Sports Sci. 1999;17:231–8.

47. Weber MD, Servedio FJ, Woodall WR. The effects of three modalities on delayed-onset muscle soreness. J Sports Phys Ther. 1994;20:236–42.

48. Meyler W, deJongste M, Rolf C. Clinical evaluation of pain treatment with electro-stimulation: a study on TENS in patients with different pain syndromes. Clin J Pain. 1994;10:22–7.

49. Bjordal JM, Couppe C, Chow RT, Tuner J, Ljunggren EA. A systematic review of low level laser therapy with location-specific doses for pain from chronic joint disorders. Aust J Physiother. 2003;49:107–16.

50. Tuner J, Hode L. It's all in the parameters: a critical analysis of some well-known negative studies on low-level laser therapy [comment]. J Clin Laser Med Surg. 1998;16:245–8.

51. Speed C. Therapeutic ultrasound in soft tissue lesions. Rheumatol. 2001;40:1331–6.

52. Webster D. The effect of ultrasound on wound healing [dissertation]. London: University of London; 1980.

53. Hasson S, Mundorf R, Barnes W, Williams J, Fujii M. Effect of pulsed ultrasound versus placebo on muscle soreness perception and muscular performance. Scand J Rehabil Med. 1990;22(4):199–205.

54. Stay JC, Richard MD, Draper DO, Schulthies SS, Durrant E. Pulsed ultrasound fails to diminish delayed-onset muscle soreness symptoms. J Athl Train. 1998;33(4):341–6.

55. Ciccone C, Leggin B, Callamaro J. Effects of ultrasound and trolamine salicylate phonophoresis on delayed onset muscle soreness. Phys Ther. 1991;71:666–78.

56. Gam A, Johannsen F. Ultrasound therapy in musculoskeletal disorders: a meta-analysis. Pain. 1995;63:85–91.

57. van den Bekerom MPJ, van der Windt DAWM, ter Riet G, van der Heijden GJ, Bouter LM. Therapeutic ultrasound for acute ankle sprains. Cochrane Database of Systematic Reviews. 2011; 6:CD001250. doi:10.1002/14651858.CD001250.pub2.

58. Klaiman MD, Shrader JA, Danoff JV, Hicks JE, Pesce WJ, Ferland J. Phonophoresis versus ultrasound in the treatment of common musculoskeletal conditions. Med Sci Sports Exerc. 1998;30:1349–55.

59. Nirschl RP, Rodin DM, Ochiai DH, Maartmann-Moe C. Iontophoretic administration of dexamethasone sodium phosphate for acute epicondylitis: a randomized, double-blinded, placebo-controlled study. Am J Sports Med. 2003;31:189–95.

60. Gudeman SD, Eisele SA, Heidt RS, Colosimo AJ, Stroupe AL. Treatment of plantar fasciitis by iontophoresis of 0.4% dexamethasone: a randomized, double-blind, placebo-controlled study. Am J Sports Med. 1995;25:312–6.

61. Ross CL, Harrison BS. The use of magnetic field for the reduction of inflammation: a review of the history and therapeutic results. Altern Therap. 2013;19(2):47–54.

62. Weintraub MI, Wolfe GI, Barohn RA, Cole SP, Parry GJ, Hayat G, et al. Static magnetic field therapy for symptomatic diabetic neuropathy: a randomized, double-blind, placebo-controlled trial. Arch Phys Med Rehab. 2003;84:736–46.

63. Pipitone N, Scott D. Magnetic pulse treatment for knee osteoarthritis: a randomised, double-blind, placebo-controlled study. Curr Med Res Opin. 2001;3:190–6.

64. Grahame R, Mattara L, Aoki K, Shichikawa K. A meta-analysis to compare flurbiprofen LAT to placebo in the treatment of soft tissue rheumatism [abstract]. Clin Rheumatol. 1994;13:357.

65. Krummel T, Dimitrov Y, Moulin B, Hannedouche T. Acute renal failure induced by topical ketoprofen. Br Med J. 2000;320:93.

66. Zhang W, Li Wan Po A. The effectiveness of topically applied capsaicin. Eur J Clin Pharmacol. 1994;46:517–22.

67. Cannavino C, Abrams J, Palinkas L, Saglimbeni A, Bracker MD. Efficacy of transdermal ketoprofen for delayed onset muscle soreness. Clin J Sports Med. 2003;13:200–8.

68. Tibbles PM, Edelsberg JS. Hyperbaric-oxygen therapy. N Engl J Med. 1996;334:1642.

69. Wattel F, Mathieu D, Neviere R, Bocquillon N. Acute peripheral ischaemia and compartment syndromes: a role for hyperbaric oxygenation. Anaesthesia. 1998;53 Suppl 2:63.

70. Nylander G, Lewis D, Nordstrom H, Larsson J. Reduction of postischemic edema with hyperbaric oxygen. Plast Reconstr Surg. 1985;76:596.

71. Greensmith JE. Hyperbaric oxygen therapy in extremity trauma. J Am Acad Orthop Surg. 2004;12:376.

72. Brukner P, Khan K. Clinical Sports Medicine. 3rd ed. Sydney: McGraw-Hill; 2006.

73. Bennett M, Best T, Babul S, Taunton J, Lepawsky M, Bennett M. Hyperbaric oxygen therapy for delayed onset muscle soreness and closed soft tissue injury. Cochrane Database Syst Rev. 2005;4:CD004713.

74. Borromeo CN, Ryan JL, Marchetto PA, Peterson R, Bove AA. Hyperbaric oxygen therapy for acute ankle sprains. Am J Sports Med. 1997;25(5):619–25.

75. Staples JR, Clement DB, Taunton JE, McKenzie DC. Effects of hyperbaric oxygen on a human model of injury. Am J Sports Med. 1999;27(5):600–5.

Index

Printed in the United States
By Bookmasters